THE SEARCH FOR THE LEGACY OF THE USPHS SYPHILIS STUDY AT TUSKEGEE

THE SEARCH FOR THE LEGACY OF THE USPHS SYPHILIS STUDY AT TUSKEGEE

Edited by
Ralph V. Katz
Rueben C. Warren

LEXINGTON BOOKS

A division of

ROWMAN & LITTLEFIELD PUBLISHERS, INC.

Lanham · Boulder · New York · Toronto · Plymouth, UK

Published by Lexington Books
A wholly owned subsidiary of The Rowman & Littlefield Publishing Group, Inc.
4501 Forbes Boulevard, Suite 200, Lanham, Maryland 20706
www.lexingtonbooks.com

Estover Road, Plymouth PL6 7PY, United Kingdom

British Library Cataloguing in Publication Information Available

Library of Congress Cataloging-in-Publication Data

The search for the legacy of the USPHS syphilis study at Tuskegee / edited by Ralph V.
Katz, Rueben C. Warren.
   p. ; cm.
   Includes bibliographical references and index.
   ISBN 978-0-7391-4725-2 (cloth : alk. paper) — ISBN 978-0-7391-4727-6 (ebook)
   1. Human experimentation in medicine—United States—History. 2. United States
Public Health Service. 3. Syphilis—United States—History—20th century. 4. African
Americans—Diseases—History—20th century. I. Katz, Ralph V., 1944–. II. Warren,
Rueben C.
   [DNLM: 1. United States Public Health Service. 2. Nontherapeutic Human
Experimentation—history—United States. 3. African Americans—history—
United States. 4. History, 20th Century—United States. 5. Minority Groups—United
States. 6. Research Subjects—United States. 7. Syphilis—history—United States.
8. Withholding Treatment—history—United States. W 20.55.H9]
   R853.H8S43 2011
   614.5'4720976149—dc23   2011014720

♾™ The paper used in this publication meets the minimum requirements of American
National Standard for Information Sciences—Permanence of Paper for Printed Library
Materials, ANSI/NISO Z39.48-1992.

Printed in the United States of America

To BJ, my life companion and inspiration for a near half-century, who enriches and expands me, to my son Amos, whose very presence serves me far better than he'll ever know, and to Binky, Madison, Carolyn, and Sandy . . . and especially Corinne, my Jersey City roots.

—Ralph Verne Katz

To three generations of supporters: To my mother, Bobbye L. Owens, and my aunt, Camille A. Wyatt, who taught me how to live; and Clifton O. Dummett Sr., Theodore E. Bolden and Joseph L. Henry, who taught me about the academy and how to function as a health professional. To Nagueyalti, my wife and closest friend, who helps me balance my head and my heart, and Hershell A. Warren and John E. Maupin, my brothers by birth and by choice. And to my adult children: Alkamessa, Asha, and Ali, who continue to teach me what life is all about.

—Rueben C. Warren

And jointly, to Tuskegee University for its daily—
and historic—importance in all our lives.

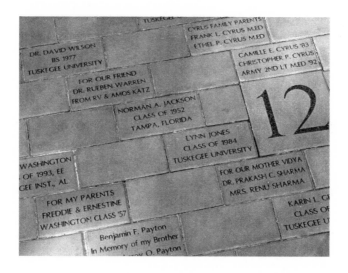

"Those who cannot remember the past are condemned to repeat it."

—George Santayana (1905), *Reason in Common Sense,*
Volume 1 of *The Life of Reason*

Contents

Foreword

The Search for the Legacy of the USPHS Syphilis Study at Tuskegee

M. Joycelyn Elders

It is a difficult thing to admit wrongdoing—especially when it consists not just of a single heinous act but rather of years and decades of continuing heinous acts that involved the faulty decisions of hundreds of people. Nevertheless, we must admit to gross wrongdoing in order to make amends for the past. We must also admit these heinous acts to those generations who come after us so that this kind of horror will not be repeated. For these reasons, I am glad to be included in the remembrance of history this book brings for this generation and those to come.

The authors of 14 reflective essays include some of the best known authors, scientists and leaders who are nationally recognized scholars whose work has focused on issues within the African American community in the context of life in America; they represent numerous fields of study and diversity of opinion that bring a broad understanding of the legacy of the Tuskegee Syphilis Study. They reflect with caring and concern on the subject, "How could this have happened and what does it mean for the present and future? " Questions they reflect on include:

1. Are minorities more reluctant to participate in biomedical research than whites?
2. Does either general awareness or detailed knowledge about the TSS affect willingness to participate in biomedical research?
3. Does awareness of the TSS and President Clinton's apology influence minority participation in biomedical research?

4. Is there a difference between minorities and whites in their ability to accurately identify the Tuskegee Syphilis Study via open-ended questions?
5. Do minorities as compared to whites believe they are more likely to be taken advantage of when they participate in research studies?

There can never be a greater scar or a more open wound for US medicine or the US Public Health Service (USPHS) than the legacy of the USPHS Syphilis Study at Tuskegee. This study has been considered arguably the most infamous biomedical research study in US history.

The study was conducted from 1932–1972 involving 399 African American men infected with syphilis in Macon County, Alabama. At the time the study was designed and implemented, there was no effective therapy for the disease. It was originally intended to study the prevalence, progression and prognosis of the disease over a limited time period.

The men were provided free medical treatment as long as they were in the study (for everything except syphilis). Also, they were provided free transportation to the research site and free meals when they arrived, and burial insurance. One only had to be poor and African American at that time to appreciate the importance of burial insurance.

The men who were the subjects of the experiment were not told they had syphilis, so they infected their wives, and their children were born with syphilis. The study's protocol expanded to study the natural progression of untreated syphilis at a time when there was no satisfactory therapy.

Finally, when penicillin was recognized as a cure for syphilis, rapid treatment centers were opened all over the country in 1947. You would think that this was a great thing for the subjects of the study. However, beginning a series of bewildering decisions, the participants of the study were prevented from having treatment for the disease that they did not even know they had, because it would interfere with the protocol of the study.

The men still were not told they had syphilis, nor were they treated for this disease once penicillin was used all over the country for a cure. When 250 of the men volunteered for military service, they were rejected due to their syphilis. Still, they were denied treatment, causing them to be denied service to their country and benefits from the GI Bill.

There were some we know of who questioned or tried to stop the study. In 1966, Peter Buxtun, a venereal disease specialist at the USPHS, reporting on the ethics of the study, was told by the Center for Disease Control (CDC) that they wanted to continue the study to completion, which would be when all subjects had died and had been autopsied. They decided to ask the American Medical Association (AMA), the white association, and the National Medical Association (NMA), the black association, to vote on the matter of ending or continuing the study at Tuskegee. Both associations voted to continue the study.

In 1968, William Carter Jenkins, an African American statistician, called for an end to the Tuskegee Study without success.

Peter Buxtun did not just drop his ethical objection to the study. In 1972, he took the story of the Tuskegee Syphilis Study to the press. Finally on July 25, 1972, Americans for the first time read in the *Washington Star* what was happening in their PHS and with the 399 untreated men with syphilis. The next day the story appeared in the *New York Times* and the day after that the study was stopped.

The USPHS knew about this experiment; they knew of the availability of penicillin and its effectiveness in the treatment of syphilis, yet no one did anything until exposed by a reporter in 1972. The fact that the study was initiated was not the problem, as no effective treatments were known at the time it was started in 1932. The problem was the decades of secrecy, denial of treatment and unethical medical behavior for which there is no excuse that is plausible. The final statistics at the time the study was stopped in 1972 (out of the 399 test subjects):

74 of the test subjects were alive
28 had died of syphilis
100 died of related complications
40 of their wives were infected
19 children were born with congenital syphilis

We must ask, "How could this happen?" Was it because adequate government controls were not in place, such as the Office for Human Research Protections (OHRPO), which was not established until after the Belmont Reports in 1979, and Institutional Review Boards (IRB) for protection of human subjects in research? Could this have happened if the race (African American), socio-economic status (poor), health literacy (uneducated), communication, or language (southern English) had been different? Was it the lack of leadership responsibility being taken by the government and those in power, or maybe all of the above? Could it happen again?

There is an old Ibo saying, "Not to know is bad; not to want to know is worse; not to hope is unthinkable; but not to care is unforgiveable. "In the Tuskegee Syphilis Study, when the experiment was begun, we did not know, and that was bad. However, as it continued after a cure was discovered, was there no one who wanted to know why the experiment was not stopped to deliver treatment? That was worse. Was there no one who insisted on offering the hope of cure to the men who were the subjects? That was unthinkable.

There apparently was no dedicated leader with the power, control or compassion who cared enough for the men and their families involved to stop the experiments and take care of the patients. This neglect on the part of the USPHS and American medicine is unforgiveable.

It is my hope that the memory of the USPHS Syphilis Study at Tuskegee never leaves us. It led to the 1979 Belmont Report, which in turn led to the OHRPO as well as to institutional review boards through which all biomedical research proposals must be passed. In any biomedical investigation or study, we must know that our first responsibility is to the patient. The patients must understand the research so that they can give informed consent. Some one individual with the power, position and knowledge must be in control. It cannot just be handed off to be managed.

For instance, the much-maligned Nurse Rivers was an excellent manager. She maintained contact with all of the participants and kept everyone informed. However, she had no control over the decisions concerning the study nor was she a physician. Investigators changed frequently with no one having a true stake in the outcome. Patients were uninformed and local physicians were being paid for a service rather than being the primary physician for the patients.

The Tuskegee Syphilis Study is part of our history that must always be remembered and faced no matter how difficult that is. We all need to know that power and government will never admit their mistakes except to another power. Only power speaks to power.

In 1997, President Bill Clinton formally apologized and held a ceremony for the Tuskegee Syphilis Study participants. He spoke eloquently: "What was done cannot be undone. But we can end the silence. We can look at you in the eye and finally say on behalf of the American people what the government did was shameful, and I am sorry. To our African American citizens, I'm sorry that your federal government orchestrated a study so clearly racist."

Neither the AMA nor the NMA has yet issued official apologies for their part in the Tuskegee Syphilis Study.

No one individual, patient, nurse investigator or scientist can be called upon to present the whole story as it actually happened. However, each of us can react, as we understand it to make certain that it never happens again.

The recruitment of minority subjects into proposed biomedical research studies have been complicated by several factors. The first set of factors is the reluctance of investigators to include minorities in their research protocols over concern that they would not stick to the protocol because of lack of full understanding, failure to keep appointments, fear they may drop out before completion of the study, fear of not being able to recruit enough patients to have a racial or ethnic comparison, fear that something is metabolized differently in one race or ethnic group as compared to another. The second set of factors are due to the feelings of the patients that they are being used as guinea pigs and are not being told the true facts of what is being done and how it will affect them. There are major trust issues with African Americans as regards the health care commitment not only for biomedical research but for health care in general.

African Americans represent 13 percent of the US population but only three percent of the health care providers and an even lower representation in biomedical research, which means that there is often a lack of cultural literacy, sensitivity and competency between patient and provider. If patients do not understand what you are saying, they cannot do what you say.

We have come a very long way since this tragedy was initiated eight decades ago or even since it was publicly revealed and ended four decades ago . . . but not far enough. We no longer have segregated doctors' offices, clinics, wards or waiting rooms, but we do not have enough culturally competent providers. We have much greater health literacy, but not enough. We must insist on age-appropriate comprehensive health education for all children from kindergarten through 12th grade. We need more minorities entering into all areas of health care, from the patient to the community health worker to policy development, clinical care, research and health education.

Until we have a population that is health literate, we will remain at risk. How can a researcher get informed consent from an uninformed population?

We want to prevent the continuing tragedies related to a lack of sexual health education, such as

- more than 50 percent of the children born in America are unplanned
- 67 percent of African American children are born into fragile and single family households
- more than 50 percent of the new human immunodeficiency virus (HIV) cases are in African Americans

Yet African Americans lead all racial/ethnic groups in the incidence of sexually transmitted infections (STI) and we deny sexual health education to our young people on moral grounds. I consider it equally as tragic as the Tuskegee Study that we still allow this to go on because of our failure to educate and empower our people.

As we look into the future, I feel that the lack of comprehensive health education for all of our people will be a greater blemish on our nation's history than the Tuskegee Syphilis Study could ever be, keeping our people poor, ignorant and enslaved to second-class citizenship. We should have learned by this time that ignorance is not bliss.

This book increases our awareness that a horrible tragedy did happen to 399 African American men and their families. We must use what we have learned to prevent it from happening again. While new rules, policies, IRB and regulations are important, the most important tool we have to prevent this from happening again is education, education, education. This book informs us through the editors' carefully selected essayists. Now, we must use this information to protect, guide and inform future generations.

M. Joycelyn Elders, MD, MS (Professor Emeritus of Pediatrics and Public Health at UAMS), was the 15th US Surgeon General, serving under President Bill Clinton. She also has been the Director of the Arkansas Department of Health and president of ASTHO. She was a member of the IRB at UAMS for seven years and served on multiple NIH and FDA Advisory Committees. She is currently a member of multiple medical organizations and presently serves as co-chair of the Trojan Sexual Health Advisory Committee. She is a pediatric endocrinologist, and was a researcher primarily in the areas of growth and development and public health, with extensive publications.

Preface

Ralph V. Katz and Rueben C. Warren

The widely believed "legacy" of the Tuskegee Syphilis Study accepted that African Americans were more reluctant than whites to participate in biomedical research due to their historical involvement in—and awareness of—the infamous United States Public Health Service's Syphilis Study at Tuskegee (1932–1972). In order to study and assess the impact and implications of this legacy so that African Americans were fairly represented in clinical trials and other health-related research, Ralph Katz, one of the book's editors, sought and received National Institutes of Health (NIH) funding, as Principal Investigator, for the Tuskegee Legacy Project (TLP). This legacy was a potential and significant barrier to ensuring recruitment and participation in biomedical studies during an era when the US government was striving to ensure inclusion of all US subpopulations in health studies.

While working with the research team and publishing the study results, the lead investigator became gradually and then acutely aware that although each published paper contained accurate data, clearly presented and reasonably interpreted, the "bigger, fuller, and truer story" of the legacy of the Tuskegee Syphilis Study was simply not being properly addressed by the process of writing a series of scientific papers. This unsettling awareness was partly due to the nature of journal publishing, that is, the TLP had to break down the overall findings into modest-sized pellets of about 3,000 words (or fewer), so that the whole picture of the legacy was not coherently and comprehensively addressed. Even a reading of the entire set of seven published papers, spread over several journals, would likely fail to identify the fullest and richest story of the "legacy." Moreover, the findings of those papers clearly pointed to a conclusion at odds with what was previously accepted as the legacy of the Tuskegee Syphilis Study.

Seeing a need to explore a new approach that would, indeed, define what currently did constitute the legacy of the Tuskegee Syphilis Study, those early concerns of the TLP lead investigator—Ralph Katz—led to discussions with Rueben Warren, a longtime colleague on issues of health disparities, that in turn led to their decision in 2008 to collaborate as editors of this volume of essays. Thus our journey began with enrolling a few key essayists, moved to finding an interested publisher, and finally to completing the list of essayists who contributed to this book.

The underlying concept was straightforward: with the new evidence via the TLP Study on the legacy of the Tuskegee Syphilis Study, invite a panel of authors to write reflective essays about the legacy of this Study through their own personal and professional prism. Thereby, the editors set a wide latitude for the authors: an essay is "a short literary composition on a single subject, usually presenting the personal view of the author" and a prism is "a transparent body . . . used for separating white light passed through it into a spectrum" (*American Heritage Dictionary of the English Language*, 3d ed., 1992).

The instructions, as sent to each essayist conveyed what we sought as editors, what we asked of each essayist.

As the editors for *The Search for the Legacy of the USPHS Syphilis Study at Tuskegee*, we thank you so very much for agreeing to write a reflective essay of about 10 pages for inclusion in this book. Each essay should address one or more of the following topics: What I think today about the legacy of the U.S. Public Health Syphilis Study at Tuskegee, what I think its meaning is as regards the specific issue of willingness to participate in biomedical studies and the related issue of recruitment of African Americans (and possibly other minority groups) into biomedical studies, what I think it means regarding the broader issues of trust/ distrust of health care within the African American community, and what it means to me about as a reflection of the current racial relations within the U.S. No one essayist has to address each of the above listed topics, but collectively we hope that this group of distinguished essayists will address this range of topics for the eventual readers of this book. No essayist should feel pressed for providing answers, rather each should seek to reflect upon where we are today on this legacy that has been discussed for the past four decades.

Each essayist has been chosen for the very special prism thorough which they would view this set of questions, i.e., a clear variety of individual backgrounds including education pathways and fields of study as well as varied work and life experiences. Each essayist has also been chosen as result of the success, scholarship and preeminence they have achieved in their own careers and fields. We believe that this rich mix of essayists will best state what the legacy of the USPHS Syphilis Study at Tuskegee means today for future health care research approaches as well more broadly for our country's health.

One word about the initial concept for this book . . . and then off you go to your reading, reflecting and writing. As our research group pursued the Tuskegee Legacy Project over the past 14 years, first within an NIDCR/NIH-funded Regional Research Center for Minority Oral Health (1992–1999) and then within an NIDCR/NIH-funded Oral Health Disparities Center (2001–2009), we specifically sought to understand the influence (i.e., the so-called legacy) of the USPHS Syphilis Study at Tuskegee on the recruitment of minority subjects into proposed biomedical studies today given the national mandate in 1994 for the inclusion of minorities (and women) into all NIH-funded biomedical studies. As we wrote the Discussion Sections of our series of Tuskegee Legacy Project (TLP) articles, now numbering 14 published articles, we developed the uncomfortable feeling that—while we were fully discussing the findings of each specific article's findings—we were seemingly missing the whole story, as that likely and understandably went beyond any one of the articles.

Thus we turn to each of you to tell the story as you see it from your prism of life, with the hope that collectively the book will present the broadest truth about the legacy today. Toward that goal, we ask that each of you first read the core set of seven TLP articles that most directly addressed this issue of the legacy of the USPHS Syphilis Study at Tuskegee before you begin your reflection and writing. These seven articles present the latest findings on the legacy, and will also refresh you on the details of past findings. But having read them you are then free to do as you will with them, once you know their content.

We fully intend that you should have a wide latitude in writing your essay, once you have read these articles. Having read them, this is your essay, so you can then either choose to ignore the details in our TLP articles totally, or you can use whatever details in them that fit into your essay idea, or you can make major use of them, including totally disagreeing with the findings and/or conclusions. The goal of our book is to advance the dialogue on this critical national issue, via your respective views and voices. Be assured we seek honest, reflective thoughts and opinions, we care not whether you concur with the conclusions of the core set of TPL articles, or whether each of you concur with each other for that matter. If we all succeed in this approach, the book will prove useful as a stimulus for continuing the dialogue on this issue, hopefully in classrooms as a textbook for future students of many fields, as well in the living rooms of concerned people who simply read it for their own edification and understanding.

So—have at it!

The essays in this book present a wide variety of prisms on the "legacy"—as intended. Each of the first four essays each takes a highly personal historical perspective.

In the opening essay, Dr. Vivian Pinn recounts her childhood memories of visits to family holiday gatherings in Tuskegee, Alabama, before moving into a broad discussion of the myriad issues that swirl around the Tuskegee

Syphilis Study and concludes with thoughts on the negative—and positive—aspects of the "legacy." (Dr. Pinn is Director of the Office of Research on Women's Health at NIH.)

In the second essay, Dr. James Jones presents vignettes of three very impressive people he met while researching and writing *Bad Blood* including new historical insights into the views of Nurse Rivers, finally revealing the answer to one of the greatly debated—but hitherto unanswered—questions concerned her belief. (Dr. Jones is a historian, Distinguished Professor, Emeritus, at the University of Arkansas and author of *Bad Blood*, the initial 1981 definitive history of the Tuskegee Syphilis Study.)

In the third essay, Dr. Susan Reverby frames her essay around the concept of a "lieu de memorie" (a site of memory) reflecting how memories on what might have occurred can shape beliefs and historical understandings more than do facts, and forms a "crucial part of what is to be passed on to future generations." (Dr. Reverby is a historian, Professor of Women's and Gender Studies at Wellesley College, and author of the recently published and insightful history book, *Examining Tuskegee.*)

The next essay is by Dr. David Satcher, who explores the role that social determinants of health played in the Tuskegee Syphilis Study, its causes and its legacy, and presents detailed historical points related to the development of the Presidential Apology. (Dr. Satcher was the 16th Surgeon General of the U.S., who spoke at President Clinton's Apology for the Tuskegee Syphilis Study in 1997; he is the former Director of CDC who appointed the National Tuskegee Legacy Committee that initiated the recommendation for that apology.)

The next set of nine essays places seven essays with a wide range of conceptual frameworks within two "bookend" essays, each written by an editor of a prestigious international health journal.

In the opening bookend essay, Dr. Mary Northridge searches for the legacy by providing a very honest, if at times upsetting, tracing of the direct and indirect references to the Tuskegee Syphilis Study and issues related to racism in medicine as printed in the now 100-year-old *American Journal of Public Health.* (Dr. Northridge is Editor of the *American Journal of Public Health.*)

The other "bookend" essay is by Dr. Virginia Brennan, who searches for the legacy by exploring the influence of historical racism in the U.S. on current beliefs and attitudes in the African American community with an emphasis on the reciprocal and intimate relationship between medicine, racism, and socio-cultural history. (Dr. Brennan is Editor of the *Journal of Health Care for the Poor and Underserved.*)

The first of the seven essays within those "bookend" essays is by Dr. Ronald Braithwaite and his colleagues in HIV health disparities research, Dr. James Griffin and Dr. Mario De La Rosa. They pursue the questions of "Could it happen again?" "What would be the signs of it happening again?" and "How to prevent that?" (Dr. Braithwaite is Professor of Community Health and Preventative Medicine and Psychiatry at Morehouse School of Medicine.)

Then Dr. Luther Williams and his co-author Dr. Monique Williams, in pursuit of the legacy of the Tuskegee Syphilis Study, seek the answer to the currently unanswered, albeit critical, question of "What was the intent of investigators of that infamous 40-year study?" (Dr. Williams is Distinguished Professor of Biology, and Provost and Vice President for Academic Affairs at Tuskegee University.)

In her essay, Dr. Vickie Mays asks, and provides a surprising answer to, the key question of "Who has benefited from the perpetuation of the belief that the 'legacy' of the Tuskegee Syphilis Study has been mistrust by African Americans in biomedical research?" (Dr. Mays is Professor of Psychology and Health Services at UCLA.)

The next essay, by Dr. Giselle Corbie-Smith and her colleagues in community-based research, Dr. Malika Isler and Dr. Adebowale Odulana, frame their essay around the interwoven nature of the long history of mistrust by African Americans and the equally long history of participation in many aspects of American life by African Americans, including research participation, and provide reminders of the delicate and complex nature of those interwoven histories. (Dr. Corbie-Smith is Professor of Social Medicine and Medicine at the University of North Carolina.)

In his essay which follows, Dr. L'Heureux Lewis opens with his personal path of growing awareness and familiarity with the Tuskegee Syphilis Study, moves to broader considerations as to what it reflects about racism in our country, and presents cautions on the interpretation of the Tuskegee Legacy Project (TLP) studies due to methodological limitations of those TLP studies. (Dr. L'Heureux Lewis is Assistant Professor of Sociology and Black Studies at the City College of New York at City University of New York [CUNY] and author of the forthcoming book *Inequality in the Promised Land: New Dilemmas in Race, Education and Opportunity.*)

Dr. Harold Aubrey takes a unique approach by framing his essay within a mathematical model of his own creation, Aubrey's Triple E Triangular Model of Outcome Probabilities, that looks to quantitatively assess the impact of educational achievement and economic condition on degree of exploitation. (Dr. Aubrey is an applied statistician, now a partner in an investment firm and formerly a higher education administrator who served as a dean, assistant vice president, and an acting provost.)

The final essay in this set of seven is by Dr. Riggins Earl, who explores the difference between benevolence and beneficence, and seeks to determine whether President Clinton's Apology was an act of benevolence or beneficence . . . and the implications of that conclusion on the search for the legacy of the Tuskegee Syphilis Study. (Dr. Earl is Professor of Ethics and Theology at the Interdenominational Theological Center in Atlanta, Georgia.)

The book's concluding essay is by Dr. Rueben Warren, co-editor of this book, who is Director of the National Center for Bioethics in Research and Health Care at Tuskegee University, as created by President Clinton in his Presidential Apology at the White House in 1997. Dr. Warren writes about hope and healing in which he deconstructs the legacy of the Tuskegee Syphilis Study, including the specific language and words used, and expresses concerns over the very name used to identify that telling historical event (the USPHS Syphilis Study at Tuskegee vs. the Tuskegee Syphilis Study vs. the Tuskegee Experiment). Finally, Dr. Warren provides detailed historical insights into how the Presidential Apology came about and concludes with thoughts on the need to address America's "sin-sick soul" on its racist history if we are to achieve the social justice our country strives for, given that it is so inextricably bound to the legacy of the Tuskegee Syphilis Study.

*   *   *

As co-editors, we sought to obtain a set of essays on this elusive topic of the "legacy" of the Tuskegee Syphilis Study, a set of essays that would likely stimulate immediate thought and feelings, as well as future reflections in our readers. Each essayist was asked to "provide their own viewpoint, their own prism" to ensure that we encouraged a variety of opinions, beliefs and approaches. In asking essayists to provide their own viewpoints, we were—and remain—fully cognizant of the wisdom, and perhaps inevitable truth, contained in this description of how evolutionary psychology views the working of the human mind: "The human mind is an arguing machine, meant to deceive its holder as well as others" (Robert Wright, *The Moral Animal: Evolutionary Psychology and Everyday Life*, Pantheon Books, 1994). As we search for the legacy of the Tuskegee Syphilis Study today, we trust that the reader will find this collected set of essays to be thought-provoking, interesting, challenging and—we hope—satisfying.

Introduction

Information Stream of the USPHS Syphilis Study at Tuskegee "Legacy," 1972–2010

Ralph V. Katz

The story of the United States Public Health Service (USPHS) Syphilis Study at Tuskegee entered public awareness when the *New York Times* trumpeted on its front page: "Syphilis Victims in U.S. Study Went Untreated for 40 Years,"[1] echoed by front-page headlines across the nation's newspapers that same day.[2-6] The USPHS Syphilis Study at Tuskegee (1932–72) was an ethically corrupt, racist, and scientifically unsound study of 399 syphilitic African American male sharecroppers in Macon County, Alabama, who were followed for 40 years or until their deaths by USPHS researchers in order to observe the effects of untreated syphilis on various organ systems. It stands to this day as the most infamous biomedical research study in U.S. history.

On its first day in the glare of the national newspaper headlines, this unparalleled discovery of research abuse often shared headline space with the news of then Democratic presidential nominee George McGovern's official—albeit soon to be retracted—statement of "1000%" support for his choice of vice-presidential running mate Tom Eagleton, whose history of psychiatric counseling treatment had just been unveiled. On that day in July, the *New York Times* lead front-page story announced "Eagleton Tells of Shock Therapy on Two Occasions: Suffered Depression," and all across the U.S. this breaking political news item shared front-page status with the shocking report about the USPHS Syphilis Study at Tuskegee.[1-6]

While the various headlines of that day would rapidly become "old news," not so for the story of the USPHS Syphilis Study at Tuskegee, which revealed previously unimagined depths of governmental callous disregard for fundamental human rights enshrined by the United States Constitution. News coverage of the USPHS Syphilis Study at Tuskegee continued throughout the 1970s; no fewer than 21 separate articles appeared in the *New York Times*, detailing various aspects of this infamous study.[1,7–26]

The Information Stream which created—and then assessed—the widely believed legacy of the USPHS Syphilis Study at Tuskegee is illustrated in figure I.1. For a quarter of century after the story broke in the nation's media, the widely believed legacy was that African Americans would not participate in biomedical research studies because of the USPHS Syphilis Study at Tuskegee. However, research findings conducted in the past dozen or so years have failed to verify that legacy, that *specific* legacy, of the Tuskegee Syphilis Study. This book was conceived in light of this newly found, research-based reality about the legacy. The essays that follow are the thoughtful and insightful reflections on—or personal prisms on perceptions of—what the essayists now believe to be the legacy of the Tuskegee Syphilis Study. These carefully selected essayists are individuals who both lived with and through the times when that widely believed legacy was accepted as true and whose lives, personal and professional, have been affected by that infamous study.

Undoubtedly this Information Stream began as simple gossip once the study was initiated, likely at each of the two "working sites," i.e., locally among residents living in city of Tuskegee, Alabama, as well as among researchers and staff up at the offices of the USHPS in Washington, D.C. This Information Stream on the legacy, as shown in Figure I.1, which began with the "word-of-mouth period," is now in a "scientific inquiry period," marked by a series of formal research studies trying to document the presence, and impact, of, the USPHS Syphilis Study at Tuskegee (a.k.a. the Tuskegee Syphilis Study) on research participation by underserved minorities in the U.S.

Prior to the initiation of the current scientific inquiry period in 1997 (which began with President Clinton's Apology at the White House to the African American community in the U.S), the Information Stream went through a period of time we will refer to as the "pre–scientific inquiry information period," which initiated in 1981 with the publication of the book *Bad Blood* by James Jones, a widely read book that is regarded as the definitive history of the events associated with that infamous study. This pre–scientific inquiry information period, after a lag of a decade, provided documentary films, plays, books, conferences and even national guidelines for research . . . all focused on the events and/or the effects of the Tuskegee Syphilis Study.

The Information Stream on the legacy of the Tuskegee Syphilis Study is alive and well today as it continues to search for the living legacy of the study. In October 2010, the front page of the *New York Times* reported that the "US

Infected Guatemalans with Syphilis in '40s" and how this story intertwined with the study at Tuskegee, sharing key players as well as a shared disease and—unbelievably—even worse unethical conduct in research.[27] Most certainly, given the importance of the USPHS Syphilis Study at Tuskegee to all the people of our country, the Information Stream on its legacy will continue into the future. Defining what constitutes that legacy in light of the recent research findings will be the ongoing challenge, as America grapples—on a societal level—with the ethics, racism, multiculturalism, paternalism and health issues inherent and so intertwined in that infamous study and so relevant to our country's future.

The reality that the USPHS, a branch of the federal government charged with protecting the health of the public, was unquestionably the primary agent driving this infamous study of "untreated syphilis in the Negro male," inextricably wove this single incident of research abuse into the broader, more complex fabric of racial relations within the U.S. In 1974, the U.S. government made minor fiscal reparations to participants and/or their surviving families: $37,500 for each syphilitic survivor, $15,000 for each nonsyphilitic survivor, $15,000 for the estate of each deceased syphilitic participant, and $5,000 for the estate of each deceased nonsyphilitic participant (compare this to the plaintiffs' class action damage suit, which sought $3 million per participant).[21] While the U.S. government made these payments "in recognition of their participation and contribution" to that infamous study, no wrongdoing was admitted by the U.S. government until a quarter of century after the USPHS Syphilis Study at Tuskegee ended.

President Bill Clinton, upon entering his second term of office, made the topic of U.S. race relations a major theme of his last term in office and announced that he would initiate a national dialogue on that topic. In May 1997, as an early step in his planned "dialogue on U.S. race relations," President Clinton—speaking from the White House—issued an official governmental apology to the "survivors of that study, the families of those who did not survive that study, and to the broader African-American community," on behalf of the federal government for the role it played in devising and conducting that unethical and deceptive study.

From that signal day in the fall of 1972, the Information Stream that flowed from those startling revelations about the USPHS Syphilis Study at Tuskegee (inaccurately but nearly universally shortened and referred to as "the Tuskegee Syphilis Study") has remained in the public consciousness, not only in the United States but also in nations across the world. The study's Information Stream and its far-reaching consequences are often referred to as the legacy of the USPHS Syphilis Study at Tuskegee. This so-called legacy, as it has played out over the past four decades, is grounded in the initial—and justifiably

The Information Stream from 1972–2010
which created — and then assessed — the 'Legacy'
of the USPHS Syphilis Study at Tuskegee

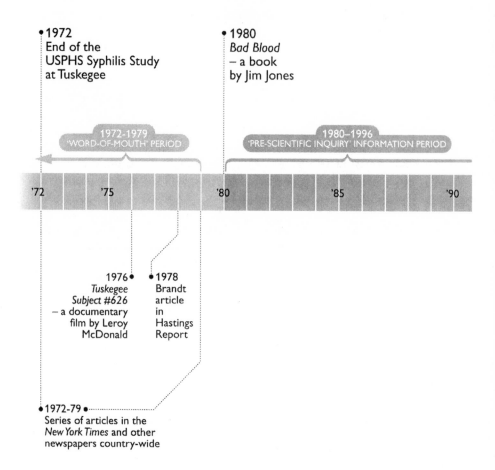

• 1972
End of the
USPHS Syphilis Study
at Tuskegee

• 1980
Bad Blood
– a book
by Jim Jones

1972–1979
'WORD-OF-MOUTH' PERIOD

1980–1996
'PRE-SCIENTIFIC INQUIRY' INFORMATION PERIOD

'72   '75   '80   '85   '90

1976 •
*Tuskegee
Subject #626*
– a documentary
film by Leroy
McDonald

• 1978
Brandt
article
in
Hastings
Report

• 1972-79 •
Series of articles in the
New York Times and other
newspapers country-wide

Created by Ralph Katz; graphic by Nigel Holmes

Figure I.1. Legacy Information Stream, created by Ralph V. Katz with graphic by Nigel Holmes.

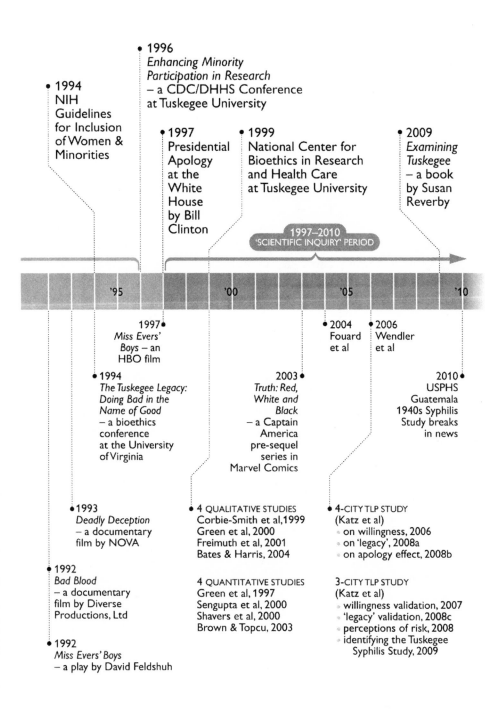

• 1994
NIH
Guidelines
for Inclusion
of Women &
Minorities

• 1996
*Enhancing Minority
Participation in Research*
– a CDC/DHHS Conference
at Tuskegee University

• 1997
Presidential
Apology
at the
White
House
by Bill
Clinton

• 1999
National Center for
Bioethics in Research
and Health Care
at Tuskegee University

• 2009
*Examining
Tuskegee*
– a book
by Susan
Reverby

1997–2010
'SCIENTIFIC INQUIRY' PERIOD

'95   '00   '05   '10

1997•
*Miss Evers'
Boys* – an
HBO film

• 2004
Fouard
et al

• 2006
Wendler
et al

• 1994
*The Tuskegee Legacy:
Doing Bad in the
Name of Good*
– a bioethics
conference
at the University
of Virginia

2003•
*Truth: Red,
White and
Black*
– a Captain
America
pre-sequel
series in
Marvel Comics

2010•
USPHS
Guatemala
1940s Syphilis
Study breaks
in news

•1993
Deadly Deception
– a documentary
film by NOVA

• 4 QUALITATIVE STUDIES
Corbie-Smith et al,1999
Green et al, 2000
Freimuth et al, 2001
Bates & Harris, 2004

• 4-CITY TLP STUDY
(Katz et al)
 ◦ on willingness, 2006
 ◦ on 'legacy', 2008a
 ◦ on apology effect, 2008b

• 1992
Bad Blood
– a documentary
film by Diverse
Productions, Ltd

4 QUANTITATIVE STUDIES
Green et al, 1997
Sengupta et al, 2000
Shavers et al, 2000
Brown & Topcu, 2003

3-CITY TLP STUDY
(Katz et al)
 ◦ willingness validation, 2007
 ◦ 'legacy' validation, 2008c
 ◦ perceptions of risk, 2008
 ◦ identifying the Tuskegee
   Syphilis Study, 2009

• 1992
Miss Evers' Boys
– a play by David Feldshuh

sustained—shock, horror, and outrage that still engulfs virtually all who hear the details of this story.

The public disgust, discourse, and debates, which in sum truly constitute the legacy of the USPHS Syphilis Study at Tuskegee, have left their own lasting footprints on a number of issues in the topography of human interactions and culture. These footprints range from the obvious and immediate (such as the unusually rapid creation of worldwide standards and enforceable policies for the protection of human research subjects) to the more subtle and sublime. For example, this Information Stream of the legacy of the USPHS Syphilis Study at Tuskegee was and remains, in its own right, a perceptible presence and force in the necessary and critical dialogue on race relations within the U.S., which, having its roots in the founding of this country, was accelerated by the photos of barking, barely restrained police dogs in Birmingham, Alabama, in the early 1960s, by raised fists at the Olympics in Mexico City in the late 1960s, and which culminated recently—and unexpectedly—in the election of the nation's first African American president.

However, over these past four decades, one of the facets of this legacy has been treated as fact—that blacks would not participate in biomedical research because of their awareness and knowledge of the USPHS Syphilis Study at Tuskegee. A series of studies conducted over the past decade offer compelling evidence to the contrary, that this interpretation of the legacy is not valid now, nor was it for at least the past decade. These studies even raise speculative questions, likely unanswerable retrospectively, as to whether that was ever the legacy of the USPHS Syphilis Study at Tuskegee, even over the first three decades after the ending of that infamous study. The purpose of this book is to continue the search for that legacy . . . and to understand ways to use that legacy for the betterment of both scientific knowledge and societal behavior.

THE WORD-OF-MOUTH PERIOD: 1972–1980

The Information Stream that issued from the USPHS Syphilis Study at Tuskegee meandered—as unplanned and unstoppable dialogue is wont to do—over the U.S. cultural landscape. Through the 1970s, this exchange of information both at the individual and community levels comprises the word-of-mouth period of the Information Stream. While this pre-1980 word-of-mouth period did include the first documentary film on the USPHS Syphilis Study at Tuskegee, *Tuskegee Subject #626*, this little-known film appears to have had virtually no impact on informing the public, as it passed virtually unnoticed in the public realm (as well as receiving highly negative critical reviews upon its release).[28-30] Equally unnoticed was an article written by Brandt for the highly regarded, but not widely circulated, *Hastings Center Report*.[31] This article, the first published article describing in detail the facts and abuses of the USPHS Syphilis Study at Tuskegee, discusses the inadequacies Brandt detected in the 1973 Final Report of the US Department of Health, Education and Welfare (HEW) investigatory panel, the Tuskegee Syphilis Study ad hoc Advisory Committee, appointed in 1972.

This arbitrarily, albeit not whimsically, labeled word-of-mouth period formally ends with the publication of the first book on the USPHS Syphilis Study at Tuskegee—Jim Jones' iconic and definitive history of this infamous study, *Bad Blood*, in 1981.[32] This is not to say that the word-of-mouth Information Stream ended with the 1970s, as the person-to-person and community-to-community exchanges continue to this day as a rich, relevant, and highly influential contributor to the critical national issues of bioethics and race relations.

THE PRE–SCIENTIFIC INQUIRY INFORMATION PERIOD: 1981–1996

Triggered by the 1981 publication of *Bad Blood*, the 1980s and 1990s provided a period that might aptly be labeled as the pre-scientific inquiry information period. This pre–scientific inquiry information period consisted of nine major identifiable elements, each of which served as "ebbing-pools" in which confusing issues and confused understandings related to this infamous study were explored by artists and intellectuals. With a gap of a decade since of the publication of Jim Jones's historical text *Bad Blood*, the 1990s was rich with ebbing-pools of thoughtful and thought-provoking reflection.

In 1992, the British group Diverse Productions Ltd released the documentary film *Bad Blood*, a riveting piece of investigative film with a superb delta blues soundtrack. That year also brought us *Miss Evers' Boys*, a play written by Dr. David Feldshuh during his training years as physician. The former was a sharp and external and insightful look at U.S. race relations that thematically used the USPHS Syphilis Study at Tuskegee as its maypole, winding the engrossing details of that infamous study around the central issue of U.S. race relations. The latter was a play that thoughtfully explored both the evil of that infamous study as well as the interpersonal tensions between its primary players. While Feldshuh centered his play around the fictional character of Miss Evers (based on the historical figure of Nurse Rivers, upon whom the success of the 1932–72 study largely depended) and her interactions with other fictional characters representing the other key historical persons, he used artistic license and stage conventions to highlight the losses suffered by the men ravaged by syphilis. To achieve this end, Feldshuh portrayed the men of the study as being keen competitive avocational dancers whose skills diminished over time due to syphilitic neuropathy affecting their legs. The HBO film of the same name, released during Black History Month in 1997, used Feldshuh's play as its base, but added a romance between Miss Evers and one of the men of the study, perhaps to further explore the interpersonal tensions, or perhaps merely to engage/entertain a wider U.S. audience. A second documentary film, *Deadly Deception*, produced by NOVA in 1993, covered largely the same territory of the earlier documentary film, *Bad Blood*, using similar interviews with many of the same players, albeit without the blues guitar used so effectively by the British filmmakers.

The next major event in this Information Stream was a one-day bioethics conference in 1994 entitled The Tuskegee Legacy: Doing Bad in the Name of Good?—sponsored jointly by two collaborating units at the University of Virginia: the Historical Books Section of the Biomedical Library (headed by Joan Echtenkamp Klein) and the Center for Bioethics (headed by Dr. John Fletcher).[33] Centered around a presentation by Jim Jones (author of *Bad Blood*) and a screening of *Bad Blood*, the day otherwise consisted of a series of papers by medical historians, medical sociologists, and bioethicists. All of these professionals spoke of the widely recognized and unfortunate—if inevitable—consequence this infamous study, namely that because of the ethical abuses perpetrated upon their community in the conducting of the USPHS Syphilis Study at Tuskegee, African Americans would not participate in biomedical studies as research subjects. In many of the talks that day, the "Tuskegee legacy" (from the title of the conference) was repeatedly defined as this unwillingness of African Americans to participate in biomedical studies as a direct result of their awareness and knowledge of that infamous study.

Interestingly, despite all the papers that were presented by academic scholars on that day, post-conference reflection on the presented papers revealed an absence of evidential citations demonstrating this legacy. Rather, all references were to this so-called fact of the legacy, including statements by virtually all speakers asserting that the African American community would not participate in biomedical research because of this infamous study. It was, apparently, a "fact," known more in the gut than in the head, since there were not any published empirical investigations. Immediately after this conference, an academic health center librarian conducted a comprehensive literature review, which confirmed the absence of evidential publications.

As an attendee at the 1994 bioethics conference, I had ample reason for concern about the implications of this legacy, as presented by the speakers. I feared the undermining effect this aspect of the legacy would have on the set of studies newly funded as part of the Northeastern Minority Oral Health Regional Research Center, for which I was the newly appointed director.[34] Funded by the National Institute for Dental and Craniofacial Research (NIDCR) at the National Institutes of Health (NIH), all the major studies in this multiyear-funded research center, which was based in Newark, NJ, focused on oral health issues that disproportionately affected African Americans, such as oral cancer, oral disease manifestations of congenital vertically transmitted HIV infection in children, and baby-bottle dental caries.

Given the potential immediate (and, presumably, strongly negative) effect such a legacy would have on subject recruitment among a largely African American community such as Newark, I planned an investigation to study this potentially disastrous so-called legacy within this potential subject pool in the Newark area. The goals were first to establish the very existence and nature of the legacy, and second, to measure the magnitude of its impact within the African American community. This was especially critical in 1994, as the NIH issued a new mandate required of all investigators funded by NIH: the Guidelines for the Inclusion of Women and Minorities in Biomedical Studies. These first two investigative steps were essential in order to develop active and successful recruitment plans to include African American subjects in the studies of this newly established Northeastern Minority Oral Health Regional Research Center.

This perceived need, i.e., to address an anticipated subject recruitment problem within an NIH-funded research center focused on the oral health issues within the African American community, led to the development of the Tuskegee Legacy Project (TLP), a line of investigation that eventually spanned a total of 14 years from conception to completion of published results. Initiated as a series of pilot studies from 1996 to 1999, the TLP created and validated the TLP Questionnaire, and eventually culminated in random-digit dial telephone interviews with more than 2,300 adult subjects (black, white and Hispanic) in seven different U.S. cities in two separate studies: the 4-City 1999–2000 TLP Study and the 3-City 2003 TLP Study. The 4-City TLP Study was funded by the NIDCR at NIH within the Northeastern Minority Oral Health Regional Research Center (1992–1999). The subsequent 3-City TLP Study was separately funded by the NIDCR at NIH within the NYU Oral Cancer RAAHP Center (*Research on Adolescent and Adult Health Promotion*), an NIDCR/NIH Oral Health Disparities Center.

Following the 1994 bioethics conference The Tuskegee Legacy: Doing Bad in the Name of Good? in 1996 the workshop Enhancing Minority Participation in Research was held at Tuskegee University, co-sponsored by the Minority Health Professions Foundation, the U.S. Centers for Disease Control and Prevention (CDC), and the Office of the DHHS Assistant Secretary for Health.[35] The major goal of this conference was to plan for an apology from the U.S. federal government to African Americans for its betrayal of the African American community. One other component of this three-day workshop conference was to have an assembly of experts on minority participation in research to review, evaluate, and critique a near-final version of the Tuskegee Legacy Project (TLP) Questionnaire, as developed within the Northeastern Minority Oral Health Regional Research Center.

The two major tangible outcomes of this tri-sponsored 1996 workshop were 1) the spontaneous creation of the National Tuskegee Legacy Committee, co-chaired by Dr. Vanessa Gamble (then a biomedical historian at the University of Wisconsin, appointed by Dr. Donna Shalala, University of Wisconsin President who in 1997 was Clinton's Secretary for the DHHS) and Dr. John Fletcher (then Director of the University of Virginia Center for Bioethics and the first official bioethicist at NIH); and 2) the report subsequently produced by that Tuskegee Syphilis Study Legacy Committee.[36] The report was produced faster than anticipated; serendipitously, Dr. Fletcher's flight home from the workshop was delayed due to inclement weather. That night he wrote the first and nearly final draft of the report, which was then edited and added to by Dr. Gamble before review by the Committee. After this review, via the who-knows-whom mechanism, the report quickly wound its way into the higher echelons of the Clinton administration, where it serendipitously harmonized with Clinton's second-term focus on race relations and constituted one of the early overt events for this focus, namely, the U.S. Presidential Apology fifteen months later, in May 1997.

As a third example of how serendipity—as is so often the case—plays a role in history, beyond supplying the TLP Questionnaire as the focal issue for one of the half-day sessions at that 1996 CDC workshop, the NIDCR/NIH-funded Northeastern Minority Oral Health Regional Research Center played a pivotal, if completely unanticipated, role in offering that workshop conference. Subsequent to planning the CDC workshop conference during the summer and early fall of 1996, the U.S. government shut down for twenty-one days (the longest ever in U.S. history), spanning mid-December 1995 to early January 1996, placing several hundred thousand nonessential federal employees on unpaid furlough.[37] During this interval, because vital tasks required attention in order to hold the workshop conference as planned in late January, it was staff and researchers from the Northeastern Minority Oral Health Regional Research Center who stepped in to carry out those essential, if merely administrative, tasks allowing the CDC workshop conference to be held as scheduled.[34]

Given that President Clinton announced early in his second term that race relations would be a major theme of his final term in office, holding this pivotal CDC workshop conference in late January 1997 ensured that the first step had been taken toward the 1997 Presidential Apology for the USPHS Syphilis

Study at Tuskegee. While this core series of events was unfolding, in February (Black History Month) 1997—just two months prior to the Presidential Apology—HBO aired its version of *Miss Evers' Boys*, based upon the 1992 play by David Feldshuh. The exquisite timing of this initial release certainly served to refresh the public's memory of this two-decades-old "piece of ancient history"—if not informing them about this misconceived and shocking experiment for the first time.

The end of the pre–scientific inquiry information period was signaled in February 1997 with the release of the HBO film and concluded in May with the Presidential Apology, delivered by Clinton at the White House. Although there was considerable discussion whether the Presidential Apology was best delivered from a meaningful site, such as Tuskegee itself, or from the prestigious setting of the White House, the deciding factor was President Clinton's relative incapacitation as he was then on crutches after the surgical repair of his knee tendon, injured after a misstep on a staircase in February.

Three following events in the Information Stream are conceptual continuations of, if not precisely chronologically included within, this pre–scientific inquiry information period. The first of these, in 1999, was the opening of the National Center for Bioethics in Research and Health Care at Tuskegee University, which, as initially proposed in the 1996 Report of the Tuskegee Legacy Committee, was then formally authorized by President Clinton in his 1997 Presidential Apology. This National Center was conceived and created to establish, out of this national tragedy, a locus of positive energy for study, discussion, and dialogue on the topic of bioethics that would serve to ensure that unethical research studies—such as the USPHS Syphilis Study at Tuskegee—would never again occur in the U.S. The second event was the publication in 2000 of the second major historical text on this topic, *Tuskegee Truths: Rethinking the Tuskegee Syphilis Study* by Susan Reverby, a historian from Wellesley College and contributor to this volume.[38]

The third and final of these post-1997 events—which conceptually closes out this pre–scientific inquiry information period—was the 2003 comic book *Truth: Red, White and Black*, published in the Captain America comic book series by Marvel Comics.[39] Published as a seven issue, pre-sequel series decades after the initial creation of Captain America, this comic book series is perhaps the most unexpected and unusual evidence of the depth of cultural influence of this "legacy" of the USPHS Syphilis Study at Tuskegee. In this series, research abuses abound in experiments, which are conducted on a black military unit to develop a "super-soldier" via an injected chemical. Once the injected chemical is perfected on this research-abused black military unit, the chemical is then used safely to create Captain America, a white super-soldier of comic book fame.

THE SCIENTIFIC INQUIRY PERIOD:
1997–2010 (AND INTO THE FUTURE)

Description of Occurrence of the Studies in the Scientific Inquiry Period

The Scientific Inquiry Period of this Information Stream begins in mid-1997. While a considerable number of pre-1997 articles, books and films had addressed the widespread belief that the USPHS Syphilis Study at Tuskegee had, in fact, had a negative effect on African Americans' willingness to participate as research subjects in biomedical studies (the infamous "legacy of the Tuskegee Syphilis Study"), all of those works were based upon the authors' own historical, artistic, intellectual, ethical, or legal perspectives and not on empirical data directly assessing the legacy—that is, no one had yet researched the validity of the widely held belief in this aspect of "the legacy." While each of these works clearly, meaningfully, and productively advanced the national dialogue both on this singularly infamous study and on the broader issue of race relations in the U.S., they neither undertook nor directly addressed an assessment of the validity of that widely held belief.

Thus, prior to 1997, there were no published, data-based research articles that had directly examined whether any differential participation of blacks or other minorities, as compared to whites, in biomedical studies was due to their awareness of the USPHS Syphilis Study at Tuskegee. A literature review on this topic, published in 2006,[40] found only eight data-based research articles that had directly addressed this question—that is, studies that had quantitative or qualitative data that assessed both awareness (general or specific) of the USPHS Syphilis Study at Tuskegee and self-reported willingness to participate in biomedical research, and all were published 1997–2004.[41–48]

B. Lee Green, currently Director of the Office for Diversity at the H. Lee Moffitt Cancer Center and Research Institute, published the first of the eight exploratory articles in 1997, based on his doctoral thesis.[45] After a two-year gap, this study was followed by the publication of seven other data-based research articles (four with qualitative data and three with quantitative data) that comprise the "early exploratory studies" of the Scientific Inquiry Period. As often is the case with new lines of inquiry, the four qualitative studies focused on defining both the language and parameters of "the legacy" as an investigative issue, while each of the four quantitative studies largely addressed only a few isolated questions within the broad range of issues to be explored, and then usually within limited population samples. For example, of the four quantitative articles, one asked subjects only about willingness to participate in AIDS research, and then only used black subjects. Another focused solely on participation in cancer clinical trials. Thus, up until 2004, the existing studies into the issue of comparative self-reported willingness of blacks and whites to participate in biomedical research in context of the USPHS Syphilis Study at Tuskegee were few in number as well as quite limited in their extent.

During this same period of 1996–99, as mentioned above, a series of pilot studies, called the Tuskegee Legacy Project, had been conducted within the Northeastern Minority Oral Health Research Center, an NIDCR/NIH Regional Research Center for Minority Oral Health. This series of pilot studies developed the extensive Tuskegee Legacy Project (TLP) Questionnaire, designed to explore a wide range of issues related an individual's willingness to participate as a research subject in biomedical studies, with the goal comparing racial and ethnic differences. As it developed over time, the TLP Questionnaire evolved into a 60-item survey instrument with two validated scales: the Likelihood of Participation (LOP) Scale measuring willingness to participate, and the Guinea Pig Fear Factor (GPFF) Scale measuring wariness about participation.

Over a four-year period, the TLP Questionnaire was administered in two large-scale, random-digit, dial-telephone interview studies. Conducted in 1999–2000, the first was the 4-City Tuskegee Legacy Project (TLP) Study, which interviewed 1,133 adult blacks, whites and Hispanics in Birmingham, AL; Hartford, CT; San Antonio, TX; and—crucially—Tuskegee, AL. Conducted in 2003, the second was the 3-City Tuskegee Legacy Project (TLP) Study, which interviewed 1,162 adult Blacks, Whites, and Hispanics in Baltimore, MD; New York City, NY; and San Juan, PR. The core findings related to assessing the validity of the widely believed legacy of TLP studies were published in a series of seven articles between 2006 and 2009.[49–55] While these seven TLP articles (see List of TLP articles in the Appendix) assessed self-reported willingness to participate, two articles in this time period by other investigators in 2004 and 2006,[56,57] added findings on the actual achieved recruitment rates by race into major national studies. Together, this set of nine studies provide the most compelling picture from the Scientific Inquiry Period of the Information Stream about the issue of willingness to participate in biomedical studies among U.S. minority groups.

The two latest major events related to the USPHS Syphilis Study at Tuskegee in the scientific inquiry period are attributable to Susan Reverby, a historian and Professor at Wellesley College. In 2009, Reverby published her book *Examining Tuskegee: The Infamous Syphilis Study and Its Legacy*, in which she examines the study and its aftermath from a wide range of perspectives.[58] If *Bad Blood* by Jim Jones, the first major book about the study by a historian, shocked and startled readers, *Examining Tuskegee* by Reverby with the perspective gained over the intervening three decades served to reflectively inform readers. In 2010, in her continuing pursuit of historical archives related to the USPHS Syphilis Study at Tuskegee, Reverby discovered a new set of documents from the 1940s about the activities of one of the lead physician-investigators from the study at Tuskegee. The documents revealed that he had, on behalf of the USPHS, previously led another unethical study on syphilis in Guatemala on military prisoners. In that 1940s study, with the cooperation of Guatemalan officials, he used several methods to infect prisoners with syphilis in order to test whether or not antibiotics would prevent infection in the prisoners. This breaking story in early October 2010, flooded the news and led to an immediate apology from the U.S. government to the Guatemalan government.[27]

Major Findings from the 17 Studies in The Scientific Inquiry Period

The major findings from the 17 studies that constitute the entire Scientific Inquiry Period, from 1997 to 2010, are most efficiently and insightfully organized and summarized under the headings of two posed questions that seek to assess the validity of the widely held "legacy" associated with the USHPS Syphilis Study at Tuskegee, namely, that blacks are more reluctant to participate in biomedical research because of their awareness of that infamous study. In logical sequence the first question is "What is the evidence that blacks are less willing to participate in biomedical research studies as compared to whites?," followed by the second question, "Is willingness to participate in biomedical research studies directly associated with awareness of the USPHS Syphilis Study at Tuskegee?"

What is the evidence that blacks are less willing to participate in biomedical research studies as compared to whites?

Of the eight early exploratory studies, only one directly addressed this question. As the four early qualitative exploratory studies used only black subjects, none of these focus group methodology studies provides a direct answer to this first question. And, in fact, only one of the four early quantitative studies (all of which used an interview questionnaire methodology) directly compared black vs. white subjects on willingness to participate and reported, based upon a single question, that blacks were twice as likely as whites to report less willingness to participate (respectively, 22% and 10%).[45]

On the other hand, the later, more definitive studies directly addressed this question and none found that blacks were less willing to participate in biomedical studies. Two of these studies, the 4-City TLP Study and the 3-City TLP Study, based their conclusions on questionnaire surveys of willingness to participate from over 2,200 subjects in seven different U.S. cities,[49–55] while the other two studies directly analyzed actual recruitment yields by race in twenty-one large-scale U.S. national studies already conducted.[56,57]

The initial 1999–2000 4-City TLP Study and the follow-up validation 3-City TLP Study in 2003 each found, by self-report, that blacks were as willing as whites to participate in biomedical studies, with only about 30 percent of either racial group indicating willingness to participate in biomedical studies, as measured by the Likelihood of Participation (LOP) Scale. On the other hand, each of these two TLP studies also found a greater—and statistically significant—wariness about participating in biomedical studies in blacks as compared to whites, as measured by the Guinea Pig Factor (GPFF) Scale. Thus while blacks were more wary about participation, they reported themselves to be equally willing to participate.

These self-reported questionnaire-based data are backed up by the two studies that directly evaluated actual enrollment rates of minorities into biomedical research studies. Both found that minorities—especially blacks and Hispanics—do enroll, proportionally, in clinical research at expected and targeted rates (as defined in the study protocols) when a reasonable effort is made to enroll minority participants. One, a report on the enrollment of minorities into the recently conducted national Women's Health Initiative Study (WHIS), stated that not only did the WHIS achieve 93 percent of its targeted minority goal, but also that the recruitment yields for black and Hispanic minority groups surpassed that of white women.[56] The other study, which directly evaluated actual enrollment rates of minorities, reviewed 20 recent large-scale U.S. studies that reported enrollment rates by race and ethnicity for over 70,000 individuals in a wide range of biomedical studies (ranging from interview studies to drug treatment and surgical trials); this study reported only very small differences in the willingness of minorities to participate in health research compared to non-Hispanic whites and concluded that "racial and ethnic minorities in the US are as willing as non-Hispanic whites to participate in health research."[57]

What is the evidence that willingness to participate in biomedical research studies is directly associated with awareness of the USPHS Syphilis Study at Tuskegee, for either blacks or whites?

Three of the four early exploratory qualitative focus group studies—all of which studied only black subjects—assessed the level of awareness of the USPHS Syphilis Study at Tuskegee and reported that awareness in blacks was "high" (remember: these were qualitative studies), but that detailed knowledge about that study was "low."[41-43] Two of these four studies concluded directly that awareness of the USPHS Syphilis Study at Tuskegee was not associated with willingness to participate among blacks,[42,44] while the other two studies made the more limited statement that subjects cited many different reasons for nonparticipation.[41,43]

Of the later, more definitive studies, only the two TLP studies directly addressed this question, and the findings of the 1999–2000 4-City TLP Study were almost exactly replicated in the follow-up 2003 3-City TLP Study.[48,54] While these studies found that while blacks were more likely to be aware of (i.e., "having ever heard of") the USPHS Syphilis Study at Tuskegee (about 75% for blacks vs. about 55% for whites and about 25% for Hispanics), no association was detected between awareness of this infamous study and willingness to participate in biomedical studies within any racial or ethnic group. As for having detailed knowledge—compared with the previously discussed "general awareness"—of the USPHS Syphilis Study at Tuskegee, both blacks and whites demonstrated very low levels of detailed knowledge, with both racial groups having mean scores of fewer than two correct answers on a seven-item Facts & Myth Quiz about that infamous study.[52]

SUMMARY OF THE EVIDENCE

The evidence from the Scientific Inquiry Period from 1997 to 2010—both the eight early exploratory studies and the nine later definitive studies—convincingly and uniformly lead to the conclusions that: 1) blacks are equally as willing as whites to participate in biomedical research, and 2) there is no association today between awareness of the USPHS Syphilis Study at Tuskegee and willingness to participate in biomedical studies, for either blacks or whites. The early clues were detected relatively consistently in those eight early studies, with the definitive findings then provided, again consistently, across the seven later studies of the scientific inquiry period.

OVERALL CONCLUSIONS

The Information Stream began with the breaking nationwide headline news in July 1972, exposing the USPHS Syphilis Study at Tuskegee, and its legacy thereafter shaping the national dialogue on the potential impact of this infamous study on the willingness of African Americans and other minorities to participate in biomedical studies. During the word-of-mouth period from 1972 to 1980, information about the study and its consequences was exchanged mainly via newspapers or by person-to-person dialogue. After the 1981 publication of *Bad Blood* by Jim Jones, the definitive history of this infamous study, during nearly two decades—referred to as the pre–scientific inquiry information period—the dialogue was driven by a series of documentary films, plays, books, and conferences, and culminated in the 1997 Presidential Apology by Bill Clinton.

Thus, for a quarter of a century, this Information Stream focused on exploring the magnitude of the impact of this legacy. With the start of the scientific inquiry period in 1997, the dialogue expanded to include a probing assessment of whether, in point of fact, this widely believed legacy was fully valid, or indeed even existed. This expansion of the dialogue, while undoubtedly inevitable in the natural unfolding of human curiosity on this issue, was likely triggered in the mid-1990s by the 1994 NIH Guidelines for the Inclusion of Women and Minorities in Research. These guidelines, legislated by Congress to ensure that NIH-funded studies would provide relevant health information on all U.S. citizens (and not just on white males), both forced the issue of inclusion for all investigators as they planned and conducted their new studies and provided other investigators with an independent central research question, worthy of its own study. Out of the latter group of investigators came the players who led the studies that constitute the Scientific Inquiry Period of 1997 to 2010.

The overall conclusion from the overwhelming evidence is that African Americans are as willing as any other racial or ethnic group to participate fully in biomedical research. This finding seems to echo how African Americans have participated in the wider arena of life in the United States throughout this country's history. As a community, African Americans continuously demonstrate a willingness to participate and serve, but never without an intelligent wariness borne of the daily realities of being an African American in the United States. The history of the African American community in the U.S. is largely one of great patience with the persistent and institutionalized racism imposed by the white majority. Perhaps this patience is based in a sustained (and likely religious-based) belief by African Americans that eventually, in time, the whites will "get over—and beyond—it."

Nevertheless, there is a continued need for sustained community- and research-based dialogue to ensure that the past low levels of participation in biomedical research by minorities remain, in fact, a phenomenon of the past if we are to have health data that pertain to all U.S. citizens. Assured by the recently obtained evidence of self-reported willingness to participate, as well as by evidence of successful minority recruitment yields when active and targeted recruitment plans are utilized, researchers can approach planning and conducting future studies not only with high hopes, but also with high realistic expectations to enroll a diverse sample of subjects. Clearly this is a marked advance over the earlier days of this dialogue, when the historical—and burdensome—barrier of the widely accepted legacy of the USPHS Syphilis Study at Tuskegee (i.e., that blacks would not participate in biomedical research because of their awareness and knowledge of that infamous study) seemed insurmountable, possibly without solution.

The evidence from the Scientific Inquiry Period of the Information Stream on the USPHS Syphilis Study at Tuskegee (1997–2010) clearly shows that this so-called legacy is not directly influential today, nor has it been for the last decade. This clarification of the legacy allows scientific researchers and potential research subjects to move forward toward the necessary and legitimate goal of realizing diverse samples of subjects in biomedical studies. Moreover, this clarification encourages further exploration of what precisely is the legacy of the USHPS Syphilis Study at Tuskegee.

Ralph V. Katz, DMD, MPH, PhD (Professor and Chair, Department of Epidemiology & Health Promotion, NYU College of Dentistry), an epidemiologist who has focused on oral diseases and health disparities, has led the Tuskegee Legacy Project research study team since its inception 1997. He served as the Director of two NIH-funded oral health research centers focused on health disparities and minority health between 1992–2009. Having served on the National Legacy Committee which initiated the formal request for a Presidential apology, he was an invitee to the White House by President Clinton for the May 1997 Presidential Apology for the Tuskegee Syphilis Study.

NOTES

1. *New York Times*, "Syphilis Victims in U.S. Study Went Untreated for 40 Years" and "Eagleton Tells of Shock Therapy on Two Occasions" pg 1, July 26, 1972.

2. *Press-Courier* (Oxnard, CA), "Withholding of Aid to Syphilics Probed" and "Telegrams Urge Eagleton Ouster," pg. 1, July 26, 1972.

3. *Albuquerque Journal* (Albuquerque, NM), "Victims of Syphilis Are Guinea Pigs" and "Eagleton Reveals History of Psychiatrists' Care," pg 1, July 26, 1972.

4. The *Daily Tribune* (Wisconsin Rapids, WI), "Public Health Sevice has been letting human 'guinea pigs' die" and "McGovern urged to dump Eagleton; says he won't," pg 1, July 26, 1972.

5. The *Anniston Star* (Anniston, AL), "Syphilis Study being probed" and "Eagleton offers to quit campaign," pg 1, July 26, 1972.

6. The *Titusville Herald* (Titusville, PA), "Syphilis Study Revealed 'Moral Nightmare'" and "Democrat VP Candidate Admits Treatment for Nervous Problem," pg 1, July 26, 1972.

7. *New York Times*, "Survivor of '32 Syphilis Study Recalls a Diagnosis," July 27, 1972.

8. *New York Times*, "Ex-Chief Defends Syphilis Project," July 28, 1972.

9. *New York Times*, "Deadline Near to Collect Syphilis Study Payments," July 29, 1972.

10. *New York Times*, "Morality: All in The Name of Science," July 30, 1972.

11. *New York Times*, "Aide Questioned Syphilis Study," August 9, 1972.

12. *New York Times*, "H.E.W. Will Study Syphilis Project," August 25, 1972.

13. *New York Times*, "At Least 28 Died in Syphilis Study," September 12, 1972.

14. *New York Times*, "Syphilis Study Went On After Its Apparent Success," September 13, 1972.

15. *New York Times*, "Regulation Urged in Human Testing," March 21, 1973.

16. *New York Times*, "Medical Care Offer Is Accepted by 77 in '32 Syphilis Study," May 9 1973.

17. *New York Times*, "U.S. Syphilis Study Called 'Ethically Unjustified," June 13, 1973.

18. *New York Times*, "Medical Experiments: Playing God: Necessary and Fearful," July 15, 1973.

19. *New York Times*, "New Rules Spark Controversy," April 30, 1974.

20. *New York Times*, "Tuskegee Dispute Near Settlement," December 15, 1974.

21. *New York Times*, "Blacks in U.S. Syphilis Program Settle Their Suit Out of Court," December 17, 1974.

22. *New York Times*, "Plaintiffs Are Narrowed In Syphilis Research Suit," July 14, 1972.

23. *New York Times*, "2 Black Neurosurgeons Defend Bahavor-Altering Operations," January 8, 1976.

24. *New York Times*, "Syphilis Suit Fees Are Over $1 Million," January 26, 1976.

25. *New York Times*, "Around the Nation: New Extension Is Granted In Syphilis Study Claims," December 19, 1979.

26. *New York Times*, "16 in Old Syphilis Study Missing After Five Years," December 9, 1979.

27. *New York Times*, "US Infected Guatemalans With Syphilis in '40s," October 2, 2010.

28. Guide to the Papers of the Capri Community Film Society, Capri Community Film Society Papers, Auburn University Montgomery Library, Archives & Special Collections, Initial Accession 1991, pg 17.

29. *New York Times*, Going Out Guide: Cinema Pot Pourri, Sept 15, 1976.

30. *New York Times*, "Screen: 2 Poor Documentaries: Medical Project and Poverty are Topics at Whitney," Sept 22, 1976.

31. Brandt, A. M. Racism and Research: The Case of the Tuskegee Syphilis Study, *The Hastings Center Report*, 8(6):21–29, 1978.

32. Jones, J. H. *Bad Blood: the Tuskegee syphilis experiment*. New York: Free Press, 1981.

33. University of Virginia Bioethics Conference, "The Legacy of the Tuskegee Syphilis Study: Doing Bad in the Name of Good," UVA Center for Bioethics and UVA Library Historical Collection Section, 1994..

34. Katz R. V., Kegeles S. S., Green B. L., Kressin N. R., James S. A., and Claudio, C. The Tuskegee Legacy Project: history, preliminary scientific findings and unanticipated societal benefits, *Dent Clin of North America* 47(1):1–19, 2003.

35. Tuskegee Syphilis Study Legacy Committee. CDC Workshop on "Enhancing Minority Participation in Research and Other Programs Sponsored by the US DHHS," held at Tuskegee University, Jan. 1996.

36. Gamble V. N., and Fletcher J. C. Chapter X. Tuskegee Syphilis Study Legacy Committee Report of 1996. In Reverby, S. M., ed., *Tuskegee's Truths: Rethinking the Tuskegee Syphilis Study*. Chapel Hill and London: University of North Carolina Press, 2000.

37. CRS Report for Congress on Shutdown of the Federal Government: Causes, Effects, and Process, http://www.ncseonline.org/nle/crsreports/government/gov-26. cfm (last accessed on January 23 2011) at www.rules.house.gov/archives/98-944.pdf.

38. Reverby, S. M. (ed). *Tuskegee's Truths: Rethinking the Tuskegee Syphilis Study.* University of North Carolina Press, 2000.

39. Morales, R., and Baker, K. *Truth: Red, White and Black,* Vol. I–VII, a pre-sequel to the Captain America series. Marvel Comics, January–July 2003.

40. McCallum J. M., Arekere D. M., Green B. L., et al. Awareness and knowledge of the US Public Health Syphilis Study at Tuskegee: Implications for biomedical research. *J Health Care Poor Underserved.* 2006, 17:716–733.

41. Corbie-Smith, G., Thomas S. B., Williams, M. V., et al. Attitudes and beliefs of African Americans toward participation in medical research. *Journal of General Internal Medicine* 1999, 14:537–546.

42. Green B. L., Partridge, E. E., Fouad, M. N., et al. African-Americans' attitudes regarding cancer clinical trials and research studies: results from focus group methodology. *Ethnicity & Disease* 2000, 10(1):76–86.

43. Freimuth V. S., Quinn, S. C., Thomas S. B., et al. African Americans' views on research and the Tuskegee Syphilis Study. *Social Science and Medicine* 2001, 52:797–808.

44. Bates B. R., and Harris T. M. The Tuskegee Study of untreated syphilis and public perceptions of biomedical research: a focus group study. *Journal of National Medical Association* 2004, 96(8):1051–64.

45. Green B. L., Maisiak R., and Wang M. Q. Participation in health education, health promotion, and health research by African Americans: Effects of the Tuskegee Syphilis Experiment. *Journal of Health Education.* 1997, 28(4):196–201.

46. Sengupta S., Strauss R. P., DeVellis R., et al. Factors affecting African-American participation in AIDS research. *Journal of Acquired Immune-Deficiency Syndrome* 2000, 24(3):275–284.

47. Shavers, V. L., Lynch, C. F., and Burmeister, L. F. Knowledge of the Tuskegee Study and its impact on willingness to participate in medical research studies. *Journal of the National Medical Association* 2000, 92(12):563–72.

48. Brown, D. R., and Topcu, M. Willingness to participate in clinical treatment research among older African Americans and Whites. *The Gerontologist* 2003, 43(1):62–72.

49. Katz, R. V., Kegeles, S. S., Kressin, N. R., Green, B. L., Wang, M. Q., Russell, S. L., and Claudio, C. The Tuskegee Legacy Project: Willingness of Minorities to Participate in Biomedical Research *J Health Care for the Poor and Underserved* 2006, 17:698–715.

50. Katz, R. V., Green, B. L., Kressin, N. R., Claudio, C., Wang, M. Q., Russell, and S. L. Willingness of Minorities to Participate in Biomedical Studies: confirmatory findings from a follow-up study using the Tuskegee Legacy Project Questionnaire. *J Natl Med Assoc.* 2007, 99(9): 1050–62.

51. Katz, R. V., Kegeles, S. S., Kressin, N. R., James, S. A., Green, B. L., Wang, M. Q., Russell, S. L., and Claudio, C. Awareness of the USPHS Syphilis Study at

Tuskegee and the U.S. Presidential Apology and Their Influence on Minority Participation in Biomedical Research *Am J Pub Health.* 2008, 98:1137–1147.

52. Katz, R. V., Green, B. L., Kressin, N. R., Kegeles, S. S., Wang, M. Q., James, S. A., Russell, S. L., Claudio, C., and McCallum, J. The Legacy of the Tuskegee Syphilis Study: Its Impact on Willingness to Participate in Biomedical Research Studies. *J Health Care for the Poor and Underserved.* 2008, 19:1169–1181.

53. Katz, R. V., Green, B. L., Kressin, N. R., James, S. A., Claudio, C., Wang, M. Q., and Russell, S. L. Exploring the legacy of the Tuskegee Syphilis Study: A follow-up study from the Tuskegee Legacy Project. *J Natl Med Assoc.* Feb. 2008, 101(2):179–183.

54. Katz, R. V., Wang, M. Q., Green, B. L., Kressin, N. R., Claudio, C., Russell, S. L., and Sommervil, C. Participation in Biomedical Research Studies and Cancer Screenings: Perceptions of Risks to Minorities Compared with Whites, *Cancer Control.* Oct. 2008, 15(4):344–351.

55. Katz, R. V., Jean-Charles, G., Green, B. L., Kressin, N. R., Claudio, C., Wang, M. Q., Russell, S. L., and Outlaw J. Identifying the Tuskegee Syphilis Study: Implications of results from recall and recognition questions. *BMC Pub Hlth,* 2009, 9:468 doi:10.1186/1471-2458-9-468.

56. Fouad, M. N., Corbie-Smith, G., Curb, D., et al. Special Populations recruitment for the Women's Health Initiative: successes and limitations. *Controlled Clinical Trials* 2004, 25:335–352.

57. Wendler, D., Kington, R., Madans, J., et al. Are Racial and Ethnic Minorities Less Willing to Participate in Health Research? *PLoS Medicine* 2006, 3(2) e19: 1–10.

58. Reverby, S. M. *Examining Tuskegee: The Infamous Syphilis Study and Its Legacy.* The University of North Carolina Press. 2009.

Essay 1

From Exclusion to Inclusion

Participation in Biomedical Research and the Legacy of the Public Health Syphilis Study at Tuskegee

Vivian W. Pinn

Memories of my early years in Tuskegee, Alabama, are of delightful family visits, of the warm environment of the African American community there, of being on the historic Tuskegee Institute campus with folks who taught or studied there, and of my first time in a hospital operating room to witness surgery in the Veterans Administration Hospital, which I was allowed to do because I was "going to be a doctor." Contrasting reminiscences are of overnight car trips from my home in Virginia to Atlanta where we could find restrooms that were open to "colored," and then driving farther south to Tuskegee—in daylight—hoping to not experience the type of encounters too often recounted by African Americans driving through the South in those days. At that time, I was unaware of another kind of experience then being endured by hundreds of African Americans in the Tuskegee area, one far different from my early memories—the realities of the United States Public Health Syphilis Study at Tuskegee (Tuskegee Syphilis Study).

Several events mark the evolution of my awareness and focus on the Tuskegee Syphilis Study. First, of course, was the news coverage about this study in 1972. I was co–principal investigator for an ongoing multisite clinical study, and the news coverage made me aware of the potential ethical and medical issues relevant to the participation of racial minorities in research. When I later became president of the National Medical Association in 1989, one of my presidential priorities was to increase the participation of minorities in clinical research. I had been briefed by some of my colleagues about suspected racial differences in the effects of cardiovascular drugs and the lack of testing of these medications with African Americans for efficacy and effectiveness in this population. With these thoughts in mind, I began visiting federal agencies about the need for drug studies to be inclusive of all populations to determine if there were differences in responses, and I spoke about volunteering for clinical trials in my presidential outreach to medical and lay communities. In those activities, it was inevitable that the Tuskegee Syphilis Study often came up as a concern, and I recall my response then, as now, that it was important for "us" to know if the medications were effective in minority populations if we were to eliminate health disparities; so I would emphasize that it was essential to be part of the research that would establish standards of medical care that would be appropriate for everyone

The major significance of the Tuskegee Syphilis Study became of much more intimate concern and attention for me after I assumed the position at the National Institutes of Health as Director of the Office of Research on Women's Health (ORWH). The ORWH was established in 1990 in response to advocacy, scientific, and Congressional concerns that women had not been consistently included in clinical research funded by the NIH. A major part of the ORWH mission, as confirmed in statute in 1993, is to ensure that women will be included in clinical research studies so that sex differences in responses to interventions can be determined. The inclusion of minority men and women is integral to this concept, with the goal that research should also determine if there were racial/ethnic differences in responses.[1] NIH began to establish policies requiring the inclusion of women and minorities in research, policies that were further bolstered by the passage of the NIH Revitalization Act of 1993 (PL 103-43) with a section titled *Women and Minorities as Subjects in Clinical Research.*

ORWH, the NIH office in which I serve, has a responsibility to monitor the implementation of these inclusion policies, and make certain that these new requirements were then communicated to researchers who would apply to the NIH for grant support. As became evident when I gave talks on those policies and rules requiring inclusion in research design, policies are of little use if people refuse to participate in the research. So my efforts began to focus on women and minorities as potential volunteers in research studies. I began hearing more than ever about the reluctance of minority women to participate in clinical trials and about the negative legacy of the Tuskegee Syphilis Study that predisposed so many to distrust and fear being a part of research studies. Early in my outreach efforts, many women and African Americans raised emotional perspectives about inclusion of minorities, and some cited the study as a negative example of what happens to minorities who, if they became involved in research, became "guinea pigs." I was often countered on public programs with passionate rebuttals from others, advising women and

African Americans *not* to get involved with research because of the Tuskegee Syphilis Study. This became a challenge for the ORWH and for me personally. I began to structure my presentations to provide reassurance that there was another legacy of the Tuskegee Syphilis Study: The development of rules and regulations and processes that should protect participants in research so that research studies today would not bring harm, and the scientific, medical, and ethical importance that policies and practices that had too often resulted in exclusion of women and minorities from clinical research be supplanted by these new policies of *inclusion*, so that the results of research studies could be applied to the diversity of our population and patients with the assurance that scientific evidence confirmed their effectiveness with considerations of sex and race/ethnicity.

It became essential to understand the major causes of the reluctance to participate in studies in order to provide the research community with effective outreach ideas for recruiting and retaining diverse participants in research studies. That was two decades ago, and today we are still discovering the complexity of influences on populations regarding participation in research. The Tuskegee Syphilis Study even today is sometimes raised as a concern, but in my experience, an increased awareness of the advantages of participating in research studies has lessened the fear of participation except at times when sporadic media attention to the Tuskegee Syphilis Study again raises the specter of abuse from research.

AN UNFORTUNATE HISTORICAL LEGACY

Unethical research practices were forced on African American women and men in the United States as early as the eighteenth century and practiced throughout most of the twentieth century. The syphilis study at Tuskegee is an example among many of historic research studies that abused the rights of the study subjects (see table 1.1). In the slave era, the physician's relationship was to the slave owner, who had total control over what would happen to the slave regarding treatment, sterilization, and experimentation. In addition, common practice was for physicians to buy slaves "on whom to conduct experiments too painful, too risky, or otherwise too objectionable to inflict on whites."[2]

It is not surprising that such historical abuses would result in fear and distrust of the medical establishment and of the concept of being in a research study—the fear of being treated as a "guinea pig." Current efforts to include women and ethnic minorities in clinical research have to consider the potential negative effects of those documented abuses and whether barriers to this

Table 1.1.   Examples of Medical Experiments without Consent of Subjects

1820s–1830s	In an 1855 account (published as *Slave Life in Georgia*) told by L.A. Chamerovzow, secretary of the British and Foreign Anti-Slavery Society, an escaped slave, John Brown, describes how he was subjected to outrageously painful experiments by Dr. Thomas Hamilton of Georgia. His body's wounds gave testimony to the experimentation.[a]
1840s–	Dr. James Marion Sims gives an account of his own experimentation on slaves in *The Story of My Life*. Among his many experiments was the use of children as subjects for dangerous experiments in tetany, a neuromuscular disease characterized by convulsions and muscle spasms.[b]
1929	The Supreme Court ruled that poor women could be sterilized without their consent. Oliver Wendell Holmes wrote the rationale that stated that it was in the best interest of the state to sterilize poor women because poverty was the consequence of a person's inability to function in society due to hereditary defect.
1960s	The US government endorsed a sterilization campaign on the island of Puerto Rico.
1963	At the Jewish Chronic Disease Hospital in New York, then an affiliate of Memorial Sloan-Kettering Cancer Center, doctors injected live cancer cells into elderly patients without their consent in order to determine if cancer is infectious.[c]
1970s	Discovery of excessive rates of hysterectomies among African American women without informed consent for the purpose of sterilization, both in the North and the South, where removal of the uterus became known as "Mississippi appendectomy." Involuntary hysterectomies were also performed in Boston to provide medical residents with the opportunity to practice surgical techniques.[d]
1980s and 1990s	Pregnant African American women disproportionately underwent involuntary drug testing for cocaine which was "justified" because of the growing use of crack cocaine.[e]

[a]Harriet A. Washington, *Medical Apartheid*. New York: Doubleday, 2006, p. 52ff.

[b]Harriet A. Washington, *Medical Apartheid*. New York: Doubleday, 2006, p. 61ff

[c]Jeremy Sugarman, in *Science Meets Reality*, ORWH, NIH, p.11.

[d]Harriet A. Washington, *Medical Apartheid*. New York: Doubleday, 2006, p.204

[e]Mentioned by Judy Ann Bigby, p. 81 in *Science Meets Reality* and in H.A. Washington, *Medical Apartheid*

inclusion derive primarily from the Tuskegee Syphilis Study or if the study has become a symbol for the composite of abuses over time.

Possibly compounding the negative effects of the Tuskegee Syphilis Study by again raising the specter of abuse in government-sponsored studies is the shocking historical event discovered and reported only recently—that several hundred Guatemalans were deliberately exposed to sexually transmitted infections including syphilis in 1946–1948. The study was directed by John Cutler, later a Tuskegee investigator in the mid-1950s, with the knowledge of his superiors. This study used female sex workers infected with syphilis and inoculations of *Treponema pallidum* to infect male prison inmates. The reported primary aim of the study was to determine if penicillin, which was known by 1946 to cure syphilis, could also be used as a prophylaxis to rid the body of the infection before it established itself.[3,4] Because both the Guatemala study and the Tuskegee Syphilis Study involved syphilis and the same investigator, it is possible that distrust about research and fear of being involved in studies could arise. However, both studies were long in the past, and when the Guatemala study was recently discovered, our government officials quickly denounced the study's unethical elements and actions of the investigators. Moreover, they issued information to the public about the safeguards now in place to protect study participants today.

Will this more recent report about the Guatemala study or other disclosures in the news rekindle apprehension? A number of drugs have recently been withdrawn from the market because of their dangerous side effects and have received media attention, although these instances have more often been related to clinical use rather than clinical drug trials. But, will the composite effect be to generate a lack of confidence that treatment trials are today being conducted without ethical standards, instead of being designed to produce reliable results that will not harm or put the study participants knowingly in danger? I hope not! And I further hope that these historical unethical studies can be recognized as part of an unfortunate past that the research community now has mechanisms to prevent.

Surprisingly, it seems that not everyone, not even a majority of the US population, not even a majority of African Americans, has heard about the Tuskegee Syphilis Study. The Tuskegee Legacy Project (TLP), which conducted surveys in seven U.S. cities between 1999 and 2003, found that self-reported willingness to participate in research studies is less than 31 percent for blacks, Hispanics, and whites, with *no significant differences* in the overall adjusted scores.[5,6] However, a significant difference was found for specific questions about *circumstances* of the study, especially the questions regarding *who was conducting the* study and *what subjects were asked to do in the study*. The researchers (Katz and colleagues) conclude that willingness to participate is a complex concept.

A different kind of study, a review of 20 more recent research studies by Wendler and colleagues, found very small differences in actual consent rates of minorities (most of whom were African Americans and Hispanics in the US) participating in those studies, compared to non-Hispanic whites. The researchers conclude that these findings, based on the research enrollment decisions of over 70,000 individuals, suggest that racial and ethnic minorities in the US are as willing as non-Hispanic whites to participate in health research.[7]

How aware of the Tuskegee Syphilis Study is the population? A 2003 follow-up study by the TLP found that 89 percent or more of blacks, whites, and Puerto Rican Hispanics were *not able* to name or definitely identify the Tuskegee Syphilis Study by giving study attributes. Even when probed by a recognition question, only a minority of each racial/ethnic group (37.1%, 26.9%, and 8.6%, for blacks, whites, and PR Hispanics, respectively) was able to clearly identify the Tuskegee Syphilis Study. The researchers concluded that it is unlikely that detailed knowledge of the Tuskegee Syphilis Study has any current widespread influence on the willingness of minorities to participate in biomedical research.[8]

Furthermore, in a separate 1999–2000 four-city study on the awareness of the Tuskegee Syphilis Study and the 1997 US Presidential Apology for the Tuskegee Syphilis Study, adjusted multivariate analysis showed that, compared with whites, although blacks were nearly four times as likely to have heard of the Tuskegee Syphilis Study, and more than twice as likely to have correctly named President William Clinton as the president who made the apology, they were two to three times *more likely* to have been willing to participate in biomedical studies despite having heard about the Tuskegee Syphilis Study or the Presidential Apology. The authors suggest that these marked differences likely reflect the cultural reality in the black community, which may be more accustomed to increased risks in many socio-cultural arenas. For whites, this type of information may have been more shocking and at odds with their expectations and, thus, led to a stronger negative impact.[9]

If only small percentages of blacks and of whites know of the study and even fewer know what it was about, what exactly *is* the legacy of this and other abusive experiments in our research history and what are their significance in this new era of requirements for diversity of inclusion in research? I am concerned to think that our society might lack a social memory of history, a memory that should be passed on through generations to prevent us from repeating errors and to make us more aware of our responsibilities to strive for fairness and appropriateness in preventing and treating health problems of all populations and for respect of individual rights and protections. I am also concerned that our assumption of a strong, negative Tuskegee legacy might itself be to some degree enhancing the legacy beyond its actual current influence and that the legacy might be a significant contributor to difficulties encountered in recruiting African Americans into research studies. To what degree might we ourselves as researchers and policymakers be negative influences because of our own assumptions or practices?

This is not to deny that African Americans have a higher fear factor of research than whites do, as found in the studies cited above—and that a certain amount of that fear is attributable to a legacy of abuse and to the Tuskegee Syphilis Study itself. The TLP found that blacks are 1.8 times as likely as whites to have a higher *fear* of participation in research.[5] Why do blacks and whites have essentially equivalent rates of willingness to participate and consent to participate when the fear factor is almost double that of whites? What is behind the reluctance of whites—or anyone—to participate? Why is that percentage at only about 30 percent? Should it be higher? Should it be double? Can it be higher? Are there issues hindering 70 percent of *all* populations from participating? Or is there simply a response plateau in any community? The legacy question has to be considered in the greater context of recruitment to research in general: if the Tuskegee Syphilis Study had not occurred, would blacks, and perhaps whites, have a greater willingness to participate and actually consent to participate as volunteers in research?

FROM EXCLUSION TO PROTECTION: EXPANDED EXPECTATIONS OF INCLUSION OF HUMAN RESEARCH SUBJECTS

Thinking about the Tuskegee Syphilis Study leaves a dual perspective in my mind. There is the negative aspect related to the unnecessary and inexplicable abuse of the men who were part of that study as well as their families. The negative perspective brings regret and compassion for those men who trusted the researchers and the physicians and nurse who convinced them that by participating in that study they would receive health care and benefits. Instead, they were treated callously and not provided with correct information about what the study was doing, nor the medical care or cure for syphilis when it became available during the course of the study. I still recall the empathy with which I viewed the survivors of the study when they were brought to the White House at the time of the Clinton apology. In addition, seeing their family members there with them, and knowing that syphilis is a sexually transmitted disease, it struck me how little is known or discussed about their wives or sexual partners. That the health professionals who implemented the Tuskegee Syphilis Study did not include specific attention to those women as part of the design of the study, offering them preventive methods or treatment, is unforgivable, and this is an additional part of the negative legacy.

But there is also a positive aspect of hope because the outrage related to this study contributed to the development of protectionist policies that to this day preserve the individual rights of those who consent to be a part of any research investigation. Because of abuses from the past in the Tuskegee Syphilis Study and numerous other unfortunate examples—such as Nazi experiments and the children in the Willowbrook State School hepatitis study—there now exist policies, regulations, and oversight committees to protect women, minorities, vulnerable populations, and all individuals in clinical studies. Informed consent is required, as is protection from research risks.

Early policies were focused on exclusion for protection, especially for pregnant women, women of childbearing age, and children. However, exclusion from clinical trials has raised concerns about the possible inadequacies or dangers of clinical therapeutic interventions when they have not been tested in women, children, or minority populations. Most notable were studies of cardiovascular disease which, for the most part, were designed around white men. There were no analyses of results for relevance to women, although heart disease was and is the leading cause of death for women in the United States, and no analyses for potential differences in effectiveness of drug or device interventions in minority populations.

POLICY OF INCLUSION

In the 1980s, as desperate cancer and AIDS patients and advocates made appeals to receive experimental drugs and willingly take responsibility for the risks, and women's health advocates appealed to members of Congress to address the lack of sex differences research on conditions that affect both women and men, the perception of fairness to access became front and center in the national consciousness about research. Policies for NIH-funded studies were changed to eliminate overprotection of subjects and to require inclusion—especially of women and minorities—in order to determine if there were differences in effect based on sex (male versus female) or racial/ethnic origin.

Including populations that were formerly considered too vulnerable to participate brought the issue of *informed consent* to an even sharper focus. Today those conducting research studies must ensure that the three essential elements of the informed consent requirement are fulfilled for those they recruit: the subject must have all the relevant information, must have the capacity to give consent, and must be free from coercion. If informed consent had been the policy in years past, studies such as the Tuskegee Syphilis Study and others would never have been allowed to occur.

As a result, NIH policy now requires the inclusion of women and members of minority groups in all NIH-supported biomedical and behavioral research projects involving human subjects (see table 1.2), unless a clear and compelling rationale and justification establishes, to the satisfaction of the relevant institute/center director, that inclusion is inappropriate with respect to the health of the subjects or the purpose of the research.

THE NIH INCLUSION MANDATE

The establishment and implementation of policies for the inclusion of women and minorities in clinical research funded by the National Institutes of Health (NIH) arose from the women's health movement of the 1980s. It had become clear that the major reason for the dearth of knowledge about women's diseases and about diseases in women was the widespread exclusion of women from participation in clinical research, especially studies on conditions that affect both women and men. A legislative mandate that women and minorities must be included in clinical research was incorporated into the language of the NIH Revitalization Act of 1993, providing statutory strength to the expanded NIH requirements of inclusion. When NIH published its *Guidelines on the Inclusion of Women and Minorities as Subjects in Clinical Research* in 1994, a new era of moving from exclusion to inclusion came into effect. These guidelines reinforced NIH policy by requiring that, among other specific requirements, NIH must:

- ensure that women and members of minority groups and their subpopulations are included in all human subject research, and
- for Phase III clinical trials, ensure that women and minorities and their subpopulations must be included such that valid analysis of differences in intervention effect can be accomplished.

FROM INCLUSION TO PARTICIPATION

The importance of overcoming any lingering negative legacy of the Tuskegee Legacy Study in generating distrust of research is this: Even though policies requiring inclusion now exist, if women and minorities do not agree to participate in research, then the intent of the policies cannot be fulfilled.

Requiring that clinical research applications include previously underrepresented and less studied populations does not ensure participation in research projects. A valid scientific study design requires an adequate number of participants and the group's composite characteristics must be representative of the *prevalence* of the condition under study in the population (and not

Table 1.2. Policy and Legislative Overview of Including Minorities in Research

1947, Nuremberg Code of Ethics	A Nuremberg trial declared 23 Nazi scientists guilty of "crimes against humanity" and issued the Nuremberg Code of Ethics: a 10-point policy setting forth the ethical constraints on anyone involved in designing and conducting clinical research studies. The Code declared the fundamental and sacred dignity of the human subjects who participate in research. It established the right of persons to choose whether to participate in research.
1948, United Nations	The principles of Nuremberg were quickly embedded in the Universal Declaration of Human Rights as adopted and proclaimed by the General Assembly in the early days of the United Nations on December 10, 1948.
1966, US Public Health Service	A series of research scandals came to public attention in the United States, resulting in PHS Policy and Procedure Order 129, the first nationwide policy for the protection of human subjects issued by the US government. Order 129 was revised later in 1966, in 1967, and in 1969.
1971, Department of Health, Education, and Welfare (HEW)	HEW revised the PHS Order 129 to further safeguard against exploitation of human subjects.
1974, HEW	HEW promulgated regulations (45CFR46, May 30, 1974) for the protection of human subjects. The regulations required every institution that received an HEW research award involving human subjects to have a functioning institutional review board (IRB). The regulatory framework stimulated institutions to take the matter of protecting research subjects more seriously than before.
1975, HEW	Regulations providing additional protection for pregnant women and human fetuses. The emphasis was still on protection rather than inclusion.
1977, Food and Drug Administration (FDA)	The FDA issued a policy prohibiting pharmaceutical companies and others engaged in the testing of drugs from including pregnant women and women of childbearing potential in Phase 1 drug trials. The reasoning was that Phase 1 trials are seldom beneficial and in some cases could cause serious harm to a fetus.
1978, Belmont Report	*Ethical Principles and Guidelines for the Protection of Human Subjects of Research.* The report talks about justice in the fair distribution of the risks and benefits of research, and specifically risks to vulnerable populations: prisoners, children, pregnant women.
1986, National Institutes of Health (NIH)	NIH guidelines on the inclusion of women in clinical trials were issued as policy shifted from the exclusion of individuals for protection of at-risk populations to inclusion with preservation of policies of protection . . .

1987, NIH	NIH policy "encouraging" the inclusion of minorities is included in the NIH Guide to Grants and Contracts.
1990, GAO & NIH	The General Accounting Office Report of 1989 revealed that women were not systematically included and were, in fact, excluded from several landmark studies that affected public health. The 1986 guidelines were strengthened on the inclusion of women and minorities in clinical studies.
1990, NIH	The Office of Research on Women's health was established to ensure the inclusion of women and minorities in NIH-funded research.
1993, NIH Revitalization Act	The guidelines were revised again in response to the congressionally legislated inclusion of women and minorities as specified in the NIH Revitalization Act of 1993, PL 103-43 (FT NT). What had been NIH policy for inclusion had now become law. In a section titled "Women and Minorities as Subjects in Clinical Research" the Act requires that the director of NIH ensure that women and members of minority groups are included as subjects in each project of research. The 1993 guidelines reinforced NIH policy by requiring that NIH, among other requirements, must "Ensure that women and members of minority groups and their subpopulations are included in all human subject research. For Phase III clinical trials, ensure that women and minorities and their subpopulations must be included such that valid analysis of differences in intervention effect can be accomplished."
1994 (March), NIH policy statement in *Federal Register*	"It is the policy of NIH that women and members of minority groups . . . must be included in all NIH-supported biomedical and behavioral research projects involving human subjects, unless a clear and compelling rationale and justification establishes . . . that inclusion is inappropriate with respect to the health of the subjects or the purposes of the research . . ."
2000, GAO Report	This study confirmed that important progress has been made in the area of involving other research institutions to conduct women's health research in a way that provides meaningful results for men and women alike. However, the study also indicates that the NIH had not yet attained the goals set by Congress. In particular, additional work must be done to better implement the valid analysis requirement.
2001, IOM Study	This study entitled *Exploring the Biological Contributions for Human Health, Does Sex Matter?* also found the need for additional work in conducting women's health research that provides meaningful results for men and women alike.

determined by general census data). Recruitment efforts encounter numerous barriers and challenges of various kinds—from conceptual and enabling factors to practical and predisposing factors. For example, the underutilization of cancer screening examinations by blacks and Hispanics, as well as those with low levels of formal education, may arise from an array of factors, including limited access to medical care, low income, poor knowledge and attitudes toward the screening process, lack of a regular physician, language barriers, cultural beliefs, and competing demands of day-to-day living.[10] But often, in discussions of barriers to inclusion of minority populations, researchers and recruiters invoke the Tuskegee Syphilis Study as an assumed deterrent.

Recognizing the challenges that some researchers have experienced in complying with the NIH policy to include adequate numbers of minorities and women in their sample populations, NIH has sponsored several conferences to identify proven strategies to address them. While the barriers vary from practical daily life encumbrances to lack of understanding conceptually of the nature of research, vital for recruitment is the creation of mutual trust and respect between the research team and potential study participants. Simply put, the entire research staff needs to understand and respect the people and communities they are recruiting, and they must make the efforts that will allow individuals to understand the purpose of the study, the potential risks and benefits of participating, and the safeguards that are in place to protect every individual who would make a contribution to furthering scientific knowledge through research.

And if questions arise about the Tuskegee Syphilis Study or historical abuses, the investigators should be prepared to respond by acknowledging them with a sensitive and thorough explanation of how individuals are now protected from risks, monitored, and will be treated with dignity and confidentiality. As stated by Harriet Washington in *Medical Apartheid,* "No one can dismiss blacks' historically grounded fear of research and retain any credibility. We must acknowledge the past in order to regain trust and to seize the future."[11] The historic events can motivate us, warn us, give us cause to reflect and behave more carefully and understandingly. The TLP investigators pointed out that while they did not find a significant influence of the Tuskegee Syphilis Study per se on willingness to participate, the study does not assess the broader question of whether and how more indirect historical events influence people's willingness to participate in research.[12] Various historical experiences may merge to form distrust; for example, there may be local knowledge of a specific research institution having engaged in reprehensible practices. If distrust is an issue, it may be an issue or barrier for *all* population groups. We need then to learn how to build trust with all population groups. What is the nature of trust? What are the actions that build trust between individuals, between groups of people, with society? In my experience, explaining the importance of the need to be a part of "the answer" to questions about health and disease, and providing information about how regulations and policies for protection are now in place, have often resulted in an enthusiasm to be part of studies. Knowledge can indeed be a powerful influence!

BASIC STRATEGIES FOR OVERCOMING BARRIERS TO INCLUSION

Researchers should understand and address the reasons for possible fears or wariness of research. Fears can be generated by external events, such as news reports from other research results reporting toxicities, or increased risks or deaths from drugs that are suddenly recalled from the market. But fears can also result from just not understanding what research is or what the specific study is designed to accomplish. In addition, emotional and psychological factors can affect willingness to participate. For example, Consedine and colleagues conclude that the fear factor is a key determinant for men related to prostate cancer screenings and for women related to breast cancer screenings.[13-15] At the 2003 NIH *Science Meets Reality* conference on inclusion, a perceived risk of harm was described: "For example, individuals might believe, erroneously, that the information will be given to the government and that it would compromise their survival—economically, or in terms of their living arrangements and their welfare status."[16]

Also, wariness, or mistrust, of the medical establishment itself was reported from a study of 1,200 community residents: "38.7 percent of African Americans and 40.5 percent of Caucasians stated that they were aware of the Federal regulations for human subjects protection . . . less than 50 percent of African Americans believed that scientists follow these regulations in contrast to almost 80 percent of Caucasian respondents . . . only 43.2 percent of African Americans perceived that African Americans receive the same quality of health care as Caucasians."[17]

A clear explanation of the study, tailored to the individual, is necessary. Explaining the study during the recruitment process covers two distinct areas: the specific research study and informed consent. Both involve education of the individuals and the assumption should be that, no matter which population group, the individuals do not have a medical education and do require basic information—and in language they can understand.

Language barriers can impede the acceptance of participation as a research subject and also the acquisition of informed consent. At that same 2003 NIH *Science Meets Reality* conference, Jeremy Sugarman provided an informative illustration of the importance of language in recruiting research subjects:

"a study in which we asked 1,882 people around the country to compare different terms used for research: medical experiment, medical research, medical study, clinical investigation, and clinical trial. In 103 in-depth interviews,
we asked people what they meant by the terms 'research' and 'experiment'
. . . respondents said that research is cutting edge, the best treatment you can
have; it is what you get when you are really sick. An experiment is when they
cut you up and put things inside you, you are treated like a guinea pig, and
the doctors do not know what is happening. A study, they said, was when the
doctors and nurses get your medical records; they read about you, and they
study about your disease. People did not understand clinical investigation:
What went wrong? Who's investigating?"[18]

These words are also confusing in the informed consent process, as again
noted by Sugarman: "You can tell me all about the risk-benefits, alternatives to
participation, whom to contact if the study goes wrong, and whom to contact
about my rights as a research subject, but if you say it is a study and not research
or an experiment, people may have enrolled for the wrong reason, and they may
not show up again. This is a problem of recruitment and retention."[18]

While it is the responsibility of institutional review boards and other entities to monitor research projects for adherence to policies and regulations, the
research community and individual teams are responsible directly for protecting and promoting the interests and safety of research participants: "We
are only beginning to address the challenges of the informed consent process
in any meaningful way. . . . Some progress is being made, particularly when
Institutional Review Boards, investigators, and sponsors begin to take a more
holistic and integrated approach to informed decision making in contrast to
an exclusive focus on consent forms and documentation. Attention to this
process avoids a preconceived notion that the desired outcome of the process
is consent and instead views the goal of the process as being to help people
make an informed decision whether or not to participate."[19]

Basic lifestyle restraints can keep some individuals from participating in a
study and small incentives might make the difference in some cases. Working people usually lack flexibility in work schedules; thus, the research team
should set schedules that accommodate the subjects. Also, scheduling concerns might have economic implications. Some individuals may not be able
to cover travel costs to the research site, whether it is in the community or
at a research center. Women, or even men, might have to pay for child care
or other family care while they are at the research site. Other home or community circumstances such as poverty, sexism, racism, or violence could keep
them from feeling safe in going out to a research site. The investigator should
be mindful of these important considerations for the potential volunteer
when designing the requirements for clinical research.

In any community, the different generations have different life experiences and opportunities than those of their predecessors. The elderly in particular have experienced different personal histories than the younger generations, and these will influence what they are willing to consent to or participate in. Many older individuals may be more apt to remember the Tuskegee Syphilis Study; they may have experienced segregation, desegregation, and other societal events that have made them more cautious or requiring more proof of trustworthiness that a younger generation. It may take more time in discussion to overcome such apprehensions, but many investigators have demonstrated their success in doing so. Representatives of the minority community may be more trusting of a research project if the research team has members of their own ethnicity. Even in telephone interviews, African American interviewees have been known to ask, "Are you black?" and they have indicated that their willingness to participate further depended on their perceptions of shared ethnicity.[20] However, for successful recruitment of minorities, it is mandatory that all research team members be culturally competent. Even those of minority ethnicity may need training in gender, racial, and cultural sensitivity.

Perhaps no strategy for building trust is more effective for a research project than to partner with the community. The partnership must be one of shared responsibilities and benefits, not just an affiliation in name only with some organizations as a public relations ploy, although endorsement by trusted leaders in the community is important. Through partnerships, researchers can enhance recruitment outreach for their studies if they listen to and understand the population they want to recruit. As reported by Kwame Osei, "If African Americans understand the research and know who the researchers are, they will participate in the study."[21] Partnering with the community will build trust in another way. Communities complain that researchers come in, do and take what they need, and then disappear. This has been common, for example, with a variety of prevention programs for teenagers.[22] Communities need programs that will not only be successful for the researchers but also that will continue to provide services for the community once the research is completed. In such a partnership, after the research is finished, a plan for continuing communication with partners about the research results and applications can go far in enhancing trust of the research community.

CONCLUSION

About halfway into the 40-year duration of the Tuskegee Syphilis Study, i.e., by 1955, nearly one-third of the autopsied men had died directly of syphilis, and many of the survivors were suffering its deadliest complications. Forty wives were infected and at least nineteen children were born with syphilitic birth defects.[23] We have experienced the reality of that study, and then its incorporation into a longer and larger legacy of egregious mistreatment of nonconsenting African American subjects: a negative legacy indeed where ethical considerations are not evident. It may be too late for those who were the victims of those earlier practices, but certainly for the present and future generations, we have responded with a new reality of protection that brings hope for the future of biomedical research. Moreover, we are moving closer to achieving the worthwhile and necessary goal of diversity among research participants at a time when we are reaching out more than ever for inclusion of previously understudied groups so that the benefits of research may be applicable to all Americans.

And so we have a history that I believe, and surely hope, will not repeat itself. But there is no question that the memory of the syphilis study at Tuskegee still exists, especially for members of the minority community. Recently, while preparing this essay, at the airport in Washington, D.C., the skycap handling my bag, a young African American man, looked at my NIH identification. He then said to me: "NIH—I know about that place—that's where they treat us like guinea pigs and do experiments on us." I was rather shocked, but in the few minutes that I had before dashing to my flight, told him, "No, today we have regulations that protect us and my job is to inform people like you that things have changed and that it is important that people like you and me be a part of research so that when we see our doctors and health care providers, we can feel comfortable that our medical care will work for us, too!" I hope I left him feeling a bit more amenable to at least thinking about the value of being a part of research! I do believe that there is a new reality, but belief in awful experiences from the past can be powerful and pervasive.

Those of us who believe in the value of research and the dignity of human life and health have an obligation to ensure that there is never another study that so devalues our peoples as happened in the Tuskegee Syphilis Study. In our roles as recruiters, researchers, policymakers, community advocates, health care providers, or just private citizens, we need to be vigilant about ethics in research, not be well intentioned but mistaken as were those community health officials who convinced the men to participate in the Tuskegee Syphilis Study. We want to be sure that researchers are culturally sensitive and protective of their research participants. We need to be sure that they are forthcoming with the full truth about benefits and risks and that their subjects are fully informed when they consent and sign forms. We have learned lessons from history, and now we need to attend to the present and build trust for the future. We must work hard with our approaches to all populations to build trust, trust built on genuine respect for individuals and genuine protection of their rights and well-being. *That can be the positive legacy of the syphilis study at Tuskegee for future generations.*

Vivian W. Pinn, MD, is director of the Office of Research on Women's Health of the National Institutes of Health. Prior to NIH, she was professor and chair of Pathology at Howard University College of Medicine after faculty appointments at Tufts and Harvard medical schools. As past president of the National Medical Association, and in her role at the NIH, she has long been active in efforts to address health disparities and encourage the participation of minorities and women in research. She was invited to the White House for President Clinton's May 1997 Presidential Apology for the Tuskegee Syphilis Study.

NOTES

1. Kelty, M., Bates, A., and Pinn, V. "National Institutes of Health Policy on the Inclusion of Women and Minorities as Subjects in Clinical Research." Chapter 12, *Principles and Practice of Clinical Research, 2nd edition.* Editors: John I. Gallin, Frederick Ognibene, 2007, pp. 129–133.

2. Washington, H.A. *Medical Apartheid.* New York: Doubleday, 2006, p. 47. The book includes a bibliography of books and articles about the history, and the Introduction chapter gives specific guidance to topics covered by a number of the books.

3. Semeniuk, I. "A Shocking Discovery; Susan Reverby Describes Her Finding that Several Hundred Guatemalans Were Exposed to Syphilis by the US Public Health Service" *Nature.com,* October 4, 2010.

4. Thomas, R., and Frieden, Francis S. Collins. "Intentional Infection of Vulnerable Populations in 1946–1948," *JAMA,* November 10, 2010; Vol.304, No.18, pp. 2063–2064.

5. Katz, R.V., Kegeles, S.S., Kressin, N.R., et al. The Tuskegee Legacy Project: Willingness of Minorities to Participate in Biomedical Research. *Journal of Health Care for the Poor and Underserved* 2006, 17:698–715.

6. Katz, R.V., Green, B.L., Kressin, N.R., Claudio, C., Wang, M.Q., and Russell, S.L. Willingness of Minorities to Participate in Biomedical Studies: Confirmatory Findings from a Follow-Up Study Using the Tuskegee Legacy Project Questionnaire. *Journal of the National Medical Association* 2007, 99:1050–62.

7. Wendler, D., Kington, R., Madans, J., Wye, G.V., Christ-Schmidt, H., et al. (2006). Are Racial and Ethnic Minorities Less Willing to Participate in Health Research? *PLoS Med* 3(2): e19. doi:10.1371/journal.pmed.0030019.

8. Katz, R.V., Jean-Charles, G., Green, B.L., Kressin, N.R., Claudio, C., Wang, M.Q., Russell, S.L., and Outlaw, J. Identifying the Tuskegee Syphilis Study: implications of results from recall and recognition questions. *BMC Public Health* 2009, 9:468. doi:10 1186/1471-2458/9/468

9. Katz, R.V., Kegeles, S.S., Kressin, N.R., et al. Awareness of the Tuskegee Syphilis Study and the US Presidential Apology and Their Influence on Minority Participation in Biomedical Research. *American Journal of Public Health* 2008, 98:1137–1147.

10. Katz, R.V., Wang, M.Q., Green, B.L., Kressin, N.R., Claudio, C., Russell, S.L., and Sommervil, C. Participation in Biomedical Research Studies and Cancer Screenings: Perceptions of Risks to Minorities Compared With Whites. *Cancer Control* 2008, 15:344–351.

11. Washington, H.A. *Medical Apartheid.* New York: Doubleday, 2006, p. 396.

12. Katz, R.V., Green, B.L., Kressin, N.R., et al. The Legacy of the Tuskegee Syphilis Study: Its Impact on Willingness to Participate in Biomedical Research Studies. *J Health Care for the Poor and Underserved* 2008, 19:1169–1181.

13. Consedine, N.S., Morganstern, A.H., Kudadjie-Gyamfi, E., et al. Prostate cancer screening behavior in men from seven ethnic groups: the fear factor. *Cancer Epidemiol Biomarkers Prev.* 2006;15(2):228–237.

14. Consedine, N.S., Magai, C., and Neugut, A.I. The contribution of emotional characteristics to breast cancer screening among women from six ethnic groups. *Prev Med.* 2004;38(1):64–77.

15. Consedine, N.S., Magai, C., Krivoshekova, Y.S., et al. Fear, anxiety, worry, and breast cancer screening behavior: a critical review. *Cancer Epidemiol Biomarkers Prev.* 2004;13(4):1–10.

16. Whitfield, K. Science Meets Reality: Recruitment and Retention of Women in Clinical Studies, and the Critical Role of Relevance. Office of Research on Women's Health (NIH Pub. No. 03-5403), 2003, p. 151.

17. Brown, D. Science Meets Reality, p. 80.

18. Sugarman, J. Science Meets Reality, p. 15.

19. Koski, G. Science Meets Reality, p. 69.

20. Whitfield K., Science Meets Reality, p. 152.

21. Osei, K. Science Meets Reality, p. 48.

22. Avery, B.Y. Science Meets Reality, p. 135.

23. Washington, H.A. *Medical Apartheid.* New York: Doubleday, 2006, p. 166.

Essay 2

Of Thanks and Forgiveness

James H. Jones

I became a historian because I care about people and because I believe that history has much to teach us. Others in this volume have addressed the legacy of the Tuskegee Syphilis Study from a variety of perspectives. I, too, am concerned with the Tuskegee Syphilis Study's legacy, but my essay is deeply personal. I wish to share with readers my recollections of three people I met while I was researching and writing *Bad Blood*. Two of these individuals played important roles in the history of the Tuskegee Syphilis Study. One was not involved with the study itself but is included because he provided me with critical assistance in the writing of that history. These individuals serve to remind us that people make history, and their stories enrich our understanding of the Tuskegee Syphilis Study's legacy. Of necessity, my reflections are subjective; I make no claim to dispassionate discourse.

In 1971, I was a graduate student finishing my doctorate in American social and intellectual history at Indiana University, Bloomington, Indiana. My dissertation was on Alfred C. Kinsey, the pioneering sex researcher. Part of my work focused on the Social Hygiene Movement, the effort of reformers in the late nineteen and early twentieth centuries to abolish prostitution and treat and prevent syphilis in the United States. To learn more about the Social Hygiene Movement, I conducted research in the National Archives in Washington, D.C., where I worked in Record Group 90, which contains the records of the United States Public Health Service's Division of Venereal Disease. This is a large record group with more than 400 letter boxes, and all the materials I examined spoke either to the treatment or the prophylaxis of syphilis, with the exception of a few boxes. These contained correspondence and reports from the early to mid-1930s about a scientific study of untreated syphilis in Negro men in Macon County, Alabama, who lived in or near the county seat of Tuskegee. I remember reading through the materials and being appalled by what I saw. But, dutiful graduate student that I was, I moved on and returned to my primary focus.

The following year I learned that the Tuskegee Syphilis Study had never ended. In 1971, however, I had no idea that it was still going on. I was, after all, working in the archives, and one does not expect a study from the 1930s to continue into the 1970s.

One other fact should be noted about my first encounter with the Tuskegee Syphilis Study. During my research in Washington, D.C., I had the great pleasure of renewing my acquaintance with Albert (Al) H. Leisinger, Jr., a career civil servant who was a senior official in the National Archives. Leisinger and I had met in the fall of 1968, when I made my first research trip to the National Archives to work on a seminar paper. One of my professors had given me a letter of introduction, and Leisinger kindly took me under his wing, sharing helpful indexes and offering research tips, as he did so often to assist countless other young scholars before and after me.

In 1972, while I was finishing my doctorate at Indiana University, I received a post-doctoral fellowship at Harvard University in the Interfaculty Program in Bioethics and the History of Medicine. I was awarded the fellowship to support additional research on the Social Hygiene Movement. In August, 1972, as I was driving from Bloomington to Cambridge, Jean Heller, a highly regarded young reporter for the Associated Press, broke the Tuskegee Syphilis Study story. In a series of follow-up pieces, Heller fleshed out her exposé, and what she revealed shocked, angered and repulsed the nation.

Thanks to Heller's investigative journalism, the American public and the world learned the basic facts of the Tuskegee Syphilis Study: From 1932 down to that moment, the United States Public Health Service, working at various times with the Alabama State Department of Health, the Tuskegee Institute, the Veterans Hospital in Tuskegee, and private physicians in and around Macon County, deliberately withheld treatment from more than 400 African American men who were suffering from syphilis. Her articles revealed that the experiment was based on deceit: the physicians systematically lied to the subjects. Poorly educated sharecroppers and unskilled laborers (many were in fact unlettered), the men were easily duped into cooperating with a nontherapeutic scientific experiment they believed was a treatment heath program.

At no point, Heller explained, were the men informed that they had syphilis. Instead, the "government doctors" told them they had "bad blood," a term then used by rural African Americans to denote and explain a variety of illnesses. To deceive the men into believing that they were being treated, the "government doctors" gave them a modicum of treatment at the beginning of the study, but not nearly enough to cure them. To preserve the deception over the years that followed, the men received aspirin and iron tonic from time to time, but the "government doctors" steadfastly withheld efficacious treatment for syphilis.

After reading Heller's first article, I immediately decided to write a book on the Tuskegee Syphilis Study. In common with most Americans, I was repulsed and saddened by what she revealed, but I knew exactly where to go to find the documents that would allow me to reconstruct the experiment's origins and begin a full-scale historical investigation and analysis. Consequently, when I arrived in Cambridge, I informed the directors of the program that I was changing topics. Instead of working on the Social Hygiene Movement, I proposed to write a book on the Tuskegee Syphilis Study. Happily, the program's directors supported my decision, and I was free to pursue the quest in earnest.

Follow-up articles in the press made it clear that the task would not be easy. Within days after the story broke, the Justice Department announced that it would investigate the Tuskegee Syphilis Study to determine if any laws had been violated. As part of the investigation the Justice Department instructed the National Archives to search its records and to submit all pertinent materials to the Justice Department. In addition, the Justice Department ordered that all such materials be sequestered until its investigation and any subsequent legal proceedings were completed.

The latter directive threw up a roadblock for me and for any other investigator in search of the truth. To be candid, I was concerned that the Justice Department's investigation would be a whitewash; and, worse yet, I was fearful that the records of the Tuskegee Syphilis Study might never see the light of day once the Justice Department got its hands on them.

This was where Albert H. Leisinger, Jr., reentered the story. When I saw reports in the press about the Justice Department's involvement, I telephoned Leisinger. After informing him that I wanted to write a book on the Tuskegee Syphilis Study, I asked for his help in gaining access to the pertinent materials I had uncovered in 1971 in Record Group 90. Leisinger listened politely, as was his wont. When he spoke, however, he reminded me that the Justice Department had made a formal request for the National Archives to locate these materials and it included an order to sequester them once they had been found. What he said next surprised me: no one to date had been able to locate any materials on the Tuskegee Syphilis Study. Record Group 90, he explained, had been moved from the National Archives in Washington, D.C., to the Federal Records Center in Suitland, Maryland, and the staff in Suitland had been searching without success for days for any material pertaining to the Tuskegee

Syphilis Study. If the records were found, Leisinger stressed, they would have to be turned over immediately to the Justice Department.

I was dismayed. All I could do was speak from my heart. I shared with Leisinger my fears that the Justice Department under President Richard Nixon would whitewash the whole affair and that scholars would never be given access to the records. Then, I pleaded again for his help. He told me he would think about it, and our conversation ended.

A few hours later Leisinger called back with his answer. He told me to come to Washington as soon as possible and that everything had been arranged. Leisinger explained that he had contacted his colleagues at the Federal Records Center (several of whom had worked for him at various stages of their careers), and that they had agreed to shoot me in under the radar and let me conduct my own search in the stacks for materials relating to the Tuskegee Syphilis Study.

Then, Leisinger gave me some sage advice. Assuming I found the records, I should photocopy them and have each document marked with the official stamp of the National Archives so there would be no doubt regarding their authenticity. The latter was important, he explained, because documents bearing the official seal would be admissible as evidence in a court of law. Therefore, if the records somehow got misplaced or simply disappeared after they were turned over to the Justice Department, the copies I had in my possession could be used to reconstruct the historical record and could also be used in a court of law. Leisinger concluded by saying that after I had located and copied the documents (again, assuming that I was able to find them) the staff archivists at the Federal Records Center would "discover" that they had them and turn them over to the Justice Department.

I cannot emphasize too strongly how much I admire Albert Leisinger and his colleagues at the Federal Records Center, and how grateful I am to them. The safe thing would have been to deny my request. The Justice Department's order to sequester these materials was clear, and it took courage for them to defy those instructions by giving me access to the documents.

Still, there was no mystery why Leisinger and the others acted as they did. Leisinger was a friend to every scholar who ever darkened his door. A fierce advocate both of transparency and accountability, he believed passionately in the public's right to know the truth about matters—large or small; and he felt that he had a duty to do his part to keep the public well informed. To me the man was a hero.

True to Leisinger's assurances, his colleagues at the Federal Records Center allowed me to conduct my own search, and I will never forget my first trip back into the stacks. The space was cavernous—absolutely cavernous. Indeed, nearly a decade later when I saw Steven Spielberg's 1981 movie *Raiders of the*

Lost Ark, I smiled in recognition when the ark was crated, placed on a forklift, and stacked among tens of thousands of other crates in an enormous government warehouse, where, presumably, it would disappear forever.

After several days of digging, I found the first cache of documents, and more discoveries followed in rapid succession. Within a few weeks, I was on the road back to Cambridge, with the backseat and trunk of my car filled with primary documents on the origins and early years of the Tuskegee Syphilis Study, all carefully stamped with the seal of the National Archives, following Leisinger's instructions. A few years later I would learn how wise he truly was.

In August 1972, my fellowship ended at Harvard University, and I accepted a position at the National Endowment for the Humanities in Washington, D.C. My duties in this wonderful agency left little time for scholarship, but I devoted every spare moment to my research on the Tuskegee Syphilis Study. The story in the press had a "flash in the pan" quality about it, and the news coverage dropped off precipitously after a few weeks. Nevertheless, follow-up stories appeared from time to time, and I monitored these with great interest. One morning a brief notice caught my attention. I read that Fred Gray, an African American attorney from Tuskegee, Alabama, who had brought a class action suit for the Tuskegee Syphilis Study, was in danger of seeing his case dismissed for lack of evidence. Cryptic as it was, this article led directly to my introduction to a major player in the story and the second person whose help enabled me to write *Bad Blood*.

A little digging revealed that victims of the Tuskegee Syphilis Study were in great legal hands. Fred Gray, I learned, was a lawyer, an ordained minister of the Church of Christ and one of the first two African Americans elected to the state legislature of Alabama since Reconstruction. After working his way through Alabama State College, he earned a law degree at Case Western Reserve Law School and returned to his native Alabama, where he waged a one-man war against segregation. In 1954 he represented Rosa Parks for violating the segregated seating ordinance in Montgomery and he went on to serve as Martin Luther King's attorney during the bus boycott in the same city. Over the next two decades, Gray filed dozens of successful lawsuits dismantling segregation wherever it existed in Alabama. By so doing, he became an iconic figure in the civil rights movement in Alabama and, by extension, the nation.

This was the man who needed my help, and I was eager to give it. After reading the article, I got Gray's number from information and called him. His secretary explained that he was not available, so I left a message. Within hours, Gray returned my call. The moment we had finished exchanging introductions, I told him I had several boxes of primary documents from the National Archives that chronicled the origins and early years of the

Tuskegee Syphilis Study. I then offered to show these materials to him, and we agreed to meet posthaste.

The following morning I called my office and told my supervisor that I needed to take a vacation day for personal reasons. Then, I carried the legal boxes of documents from my study, stacked them on the dining room table, and waited. Around 10 a.m., I heard a loud knocking. I opened my front door to find a strikingly handsome man of medium height and build smiling broadly at me. After we exchanged greetings and shook hands, I invited him inside, and Fred Gray stepped into my home and into my life.

He immediately spotted the legal boxes. Without saying a word, he walked directly to my dining room table and stood by the boxes. I was only a step behind, but by the time I had pulled even Gray had helped himself to a banana from a bowl of fruit next to the boxes, peeled it, and was devouring it, all the while peering at me with eyes that said, "Come on man; let's get started." To this day, I remember thinking to myself, "I like this guy. He doesn't stand on ceremony. We are going to be friends."

I took the lid off the first box and Gray immediately plunged in. He spent the next hour or so reading documents, while I talked a mile a minute about the story the materials revealed. In addition, I pointed out that each of the documents had been stamped with the official seal of the National Archives and was therefore admissible in a court of law, a fact that delighted Gray. Then, we stood back from the treasure trove of documents and discussed what to do next. Based on the volume of materials I had found on the experiment's origins and early years, I volunteered the opinion that there had to be thousands of additional documents pertaining to the remaining decades of the experiment's history, if only we could find them.

Again, up to this point, Gray had been totally frustrated in his efforts to pry documents from the Justice Department. Every request he had made as part of the discovery process had been met with the same answer: so far as the government knew, no records were available. The documents I had found in the National Archives were a game changer. Gray told me that he would use them to pry loose the materials that had eluded him to date from the Justice Department and the Centers for Disease Control (CDC).

After explaining his strategy, Gray asked me to assist him with the research in what now promised to be a fruitful process of discovery. I agreed to do so, but not on the full-time basis he proposed. I explained to Gray that I had a professional commitment to the National Endowment for the Humanities, and that I could not take a leave of absence from these duties. The best I could do, I continued, would be to give him my weekends, my vacation days, and every other minute I could "beg, borrow, or steal" to help with the case. Gray accepted these terms, and he offered to pay for my assistance. I demurred, insisting that the all I wanted was research expenses and his promise that I would be given copies of all the materials we uncovered for the case and permission to cite them in my book. We shook hands, and the deal was struck.

Throughout 1974 and 1975, Gray worked hard to prepare for trial. Armed with the materials I provided, Gray got the Justice Department to surrender the mother lode of documents, which then were housed at the CDC in Atlanta, Georgia. He received vital assistance from Harold Edgar, a brilliant young law professor from Columbia University who worked pro bono helping him develop the legal arguments in the case. Edgar and I descended on the CDC, and where no materials were supposed to exist, we emerged with thousands of documents, which took up where the materials I had given Gray stopped. Together, the two caches chronicled the forty-year history of the Tuskegee Syphilis Study in rich detail, providing more than enough documentary evidence for Gray to support each of the charges in his lawsuit. Edgar and I also helped Gray prepare for the depositions with the key figures from the Public Health Service.

The depositions went forward, but once Gray had the goods, there was no way the Justice Department wanted to try the case. It was settled out of court. In addition to free medical care for the rest of their lives, the men and their families received a financial settlement—not as much money as Gray had hoped to get them, but enough to cushion their lives in old age.

True to his word, Gray returned my help in kind. He personally arranged for me to interview a number of his clients who were plaintiffs in the case. I am deeply grateful to Gray for this assistance, for the men he persuaded to talk with me provided some of the most poignant voices in *Bad Blood*. And despite my insistence that I did not want to be paid, Gray later sent me a check for several thousand dollars—his way of underscoring his gratitude.

But Gray was the person who deserved my thanks. During the two years that I had the privilege of working with him, I came to like, respect and admire him greatly. His legal skills left me in awe; his devotion to his clients warmed my heart, and his fierce commitment to social justice and to the rule of law inspired me. Together with so many other people whose lives he has touched, I am deeply indebted to this good and noble man. Without his help, *Bad Blood* would never have been written.

The last person I wish to discuss is Eunice Rivers Laurie (Nurse Rivers). Readers of *Bad Blood* know that Nurse Rivers (her maiden name and the name by which she was called throughout the Tuskegee Syphilis Study's forty-year history) is the only person to whom I devoted an entire chapter. What is not well known, however, is that I made three separate passes at that chapter before settling on the version I published. The first draft I wrote in anger, and the figure who emerged in these pages bore a striking resemblance to Nurse

Mildred Ratched, a.k.a. "Big Nurse," the principal antagonist, played to perfection by Louise Fletcher, in the 1975 movie *One Flew Over the Cuckoo's Nest*. In my second draft, the pendulum swung to the opposite extreme, and the Nurse Rivers I created had an aura that bought to mind Florence Nightingale. In the third and final draft, I found a resting place and made my peace with this tragic, complex, confounding and ultimately, I think, good woman.

Part of my difficulty was the fear that I had been co-opted by Nurse Rivers. For several years, she declined my numerous requests for an interview, but when she finally agreed to see me she was extraordinarily generous and helpful. We spent several days together driving around the hinterland of Tuskegee. Each turn of the road seemed to trigger a flood of memories in her, and she regaled me with stories about her life with the men. Again and again, I was struck by the genuine affection in her voice when she reminisced about "the patients" in the Tuskegee Syphilis Study. I found the whole experience profoundly unsettling, largely, I suspect, because she disabused me of many of the preconceived notions I had about her as a person and about the critical role she played in keeping the experiment going for forty years. Thus, the difficulty I experienced when I later tried to capture her and her role on paper.

On our final day together, I ended my formal interview with Nurse Rivers after several hours of intense discussion. Instead of departing promptly, however, I tarried for a time and we continued talking with my tape recorder turned off. We sat together on a couch in the living room of her modest, immaculate home. On the wall above us, hung a portrait of Martin Luther King and a framed copy of the "Florence Nightingale Pledge." As we continued talking, I got the distinct impression that Nurse Rivers did not want me to leave—that there was something else she wanted to tell me. So, I decided to revisit an important issue. On several occasions during the preceding days, Nurse River had attempted to broach a painful subject, volunteering that perhaps mistakes had been made in the Tuskegee Syphilis Study. But every time she had raised this subject, I had cut her off, explaining that it was not my role to judge. "I just want to try to understand what happened," I recall saying.

When the moment came to say good-bye and leave, I mentioned her attempts to discuss the mistakes that haunted her, apologized for the interruptions and asked her to tell me what she thought they had done wrong. For what seemed like an eternity, Nurse Rivers sat there in silence. When she spoke, her reply was heart-wrenching. Voice laden with emotion, lower lip quivering, struggling to maintain her composure, she cast her head down, closed her eyes, and sobbed, "Oh, Dr. Jones. We should have told the men they had syphilis, and God knows we should have treated them."

When she regained control of herself, Nurse Rivers opened her eyes. For the first time since we met, spoken words eluded her. She had no words. But her eyes begged for forgiveness. I could not give it because I felt too much anger toward her. So we said our good-byes, and I left without granting the absolution she wanted so badly. The year was 1977, and I never saw or spoke with Nurse Rivers again.

Because we had spoken off the record, I elected not to use her words in *Bad Blood*. Eunice Rivers Laurie died in 1986. I now feel free to share her confession with others. To my knowledge, she is the only individual among a large group with varying degrees of responsible for the Tuskegee Syphilis Study to acknowledge wrongdoing and to express remorse.

To do so took character. Nurse Rivers devoted several decades of her life to the Tuskegee Syphilis Study, only to confront the moral calamity of her actions in the end. She was a Christian woman who believed that it was her duty to perform good works. How did she feel once she finally realized that she had toiled so long and so hard on a study in which a long list of other caregivers and she had stood idle while people in her community had suffered and died because they were denied treatment for their disease? She, alone, knew the answer.

But as we reflect on the Tuskegee Syphilis Study's legacy, I think we should weigh carefully what Nurse Rivers said to me. Her lament contained more than a hint of sorrow and contrition. In the end, Nurse Rivers understood that the Tuskegee Syphilis Study was wrong, and she said so. There is no doubt in my mind that she felt remorse.

Thirty years have passed since I published *Bad Blood*, and I still have not taken my leave of Nurse Rivers. In my book's acknowledgments, I confessed that pondering her life had increased my tolerance for moral ambiguity and had helped me to understand why good people sin. To this day, she haunts me. After more than a third of a century of reflection, I pray fervently that the Tuskegee Syphilis Study's legacy will include forgiveness for Nurse Rivers.

James H. Jones, PhD (alumni distinguished professor, emeritus, University of Arkansas), is an American social and intellectual historian who specializes in the history of science and medicine. In addition to Bad Blood: The Tuskegee Syphilis Experiment, *he is the author of* Alfred C. Kinsey, A Public/Private Life. *His essays and book reviews have appeared in* The New Yorker, *the* New York Times, *the* Washington Post, *and the* Los Angeles Times. *He lives in Washington, D.C.*

Essay 3

The Tuskegee Syphilis Study as a "Site of Memory"

Susan M. Reverby

The legacy of the Tuskegee Syphilis Study is entwined in beliefs about racism and scientific/clinical hubris that are often deficient in factual understandings of the Study itself. For nearly two decades I have tried in books, articles, lectures, interviews and web-based rants to separate out *what happened* during the Study's forty years from what *has happened* in the nearly forty years since it ended. My somewhat fruitful (producing scholarship) and often fruitless (producing knowledge) efforts are telling reminders of the ways memories of what *might* have occurred shape historical understandings and contemporary beliefs.[1]

The increasingly iconic status of the Study makes it what French historian Pierre Nora calls a *lieu de memoire*, a site of memory that is not merely a physical place, monument or celebration, but rather an interaction between history and memory, an event or experience, imagined *and* factual at the same time.[2] The creation of a site of memory becomes the way in which individuals and groups in societies make meanings of their experiences and histories. "What is remembered [in this way]," African American literary scholars Geneviève Fabre and Robert O'Meally argue, can become "a crucial part of what is to be passed on to future generations."[3]

To explain the Study as a site of memory is to understand it is not just an experiment created by the U.S. Public Health Service (PHS) researchers and experienced by the men and their families in Alabama, and retold by historians and bioethicists. Rather it has become a symbolic and memorialized site that is available to give meaning to the reality of scientific endeavors, ever-present

29

racism, state power, and the experiences of those who face illness and reach for help. Clinicians and researchers cite it when they want to show their cultural competency and assumptions about the Study's affect on their African American patients or possible subjects in a clinical trial. Political actors from the left and the right call upon it to indicate knowledge of dangerous federal power. Writers in the media signal it to explain dangers for African Americans of one kind or another in contemporary times. *Saturday Night Live* had one of its characters utter "Tuskegee, Tuskegee, Tuskegee" to explain the danger of a white doctor treating a black patient.[4] Even if individuals do not know what it means or do not cite it specifically, the words "Tuskegee syphilis study" now have cultural validity and are part of the American vernacular.

These multiple usages happen, even if the details of the actual study itself are blurry, unknown or just wrong. It reminds us that what comedian/social commentator Stephen Colbert called "truthiness" and psychologist Craig Barclay labeled "true but not veridical" is what individuals—potential clinical trial subjects, clinicians, public health personnel, writers, bloggers—often believe about what happened during the Study.[5] This confusion of fact and fiction is central to the Study's legacy and creation as a site of memory, and is made in multiple communities.[6]

Misunderstandings are not just limited to those who only learn about the Study through rumor or undocumented websites.[7] As we move further and further away from an actual memory of the Study's public exposure (whether through the 1972 news accounts, the 1992–93 television documentaries on HBO and ABC, the 1997 federal apology, or the multiple re-showings of the fictionalized *Miss Evers' Boys*), the factual errors abound and serve to deepen the Study's cultural power.[8]

It is what is remembered that matters in the creation of the Study as a site of memory, not just what happened, since in our ahistorical society the spinning social amnesia takes over the actual events. The Study, as a site or story, thus overwhelms any of the historical details and its didactic usage becomes more available.[9] Its power comes *precisely* because the details are confused. Stories always seem to win over historical narratives because they appeal, in this case, to our desire to understand something about racism, medical science, and human subject protection and we fit the facts to our story-driven beliefs.[10]

JUST THE FACTS

Confusion over what actually happened is perhaps inevitable in something as long-standing and long remembered as the Study.[11] It can become a site of memory because its history is full of facts that are not simple to know. Every time I have to write about the Study, or even worse when I have to do an interview, I am reminded how difficult it is to get everything correct, especially in a few sentences. Confusion reigns in particular over how many men were in the Study, what happened to them, and to their families and is central to the power of the legacy.

Even something as basic as how many men were in the Study is bandied about. The often-repeated figure from the initial stories is 399 subjects and 201 controls that add up to 600—a horrifying yet rememberable number.[12] We also know from the reports, however, that some of the controls were shifted into the subjects' category when they developed syphilis. Exactly how many is not certain because the numbers change in the various reports— probably somewhere between 12 and 19. The numbers of those with the disease who were the "real" subjects are not so simple to fathom either. Some of the subjects who died and were autopsied did not show signs of syphilis on their bodies. They should have probably been controls, but were not placed back into the control category.

The medical records of the men are now available in the Southeast Regional National Archives in Morrow, Georgia. The best final number of the men involved I can deduce from them is 624: 427 assumed to have the disease, 185 without, and another 12 shifted from control to subject. Does it matter in the end to get the actual numbers correct? Yes, because we should know as best we can and the families should know all their names. No because the roundness of the 600 makes the number rememberable as the fact of how many controls, how many subjects, slips away, and the sense of each of the Study's men as a black "everyman" stays firmly in our minds.[13]

The morbidity and mortality that the lack of treatment caused is central, as well, to the Study's ability to be a site of memory. The disease can affect differing organs of the body and can cause other illnesses and death. Syphilis used to be called "the great imitator" because its affects mimicked numerous other diseases even when it did not cause them. Its damage to the body varied by individuals and many died with syphilis, not from it. Others suffered severe cardiovascular and neurological complications that filled them with blindness, aneurysms and pain. Despite stories to the contrary, however, not all of the men died from syphilis.

The reports and medical files reveal the damage that it is possible to acknowledge: up until the last years of the Study those who were assumed to have syphilis did much worse than the controls. Life tables created in 1955 showed that at least for the younger men in the Study, aged 20–50; those assumed to have syphilis had a 17 percent shorter life expectancy. They became sicker and died sooner (the controls on average at 70 and the untreated and inadequately treated syphilitics at 65).

The initial news stories, based on the published articles, estimated the deaths widely from 9, to 28, to 100, while other accounts circulate that make it appear as if all the men died from the disease. Given that the categories for how to report cause of death shifted over the years, the failure to have records on the men who passed away after the Study closed (74 were still alive in 1972), and the differences between the limited autopsy reports and tissue data, we will never know this number exactly. In the medical records, sixteen men have syphilis listed as the cause of death. If it was, however, the primary cause of death is not clear.[14] Even one death, of course, is too many. Yet we ought to be able to know what affect the Study had more clearly than we do and so the stories proliferate.

In Macon County itself, a father, grandfather or uncle in the Study provides many with an explanatory framework for their own family's history. The daughter of one of the men in the Study, for example, in a major newspaper interview and in open discussion, talked about remembering her father's shortness of breath caused by his untreated disease. In going through the Study's medical records, I found that this man died from lung cancer that would explain his inability to breathe. This fact helps me write a more factual history. Would it, however, change the beliefs of the family about what caused his death and their sense about how they were wronged?

Even the issue of treatment has to be considered as part of the factual confusion. The lack of intentional treatment is clear in the multiple titles of the published articles: "Untreated Syphilis in the Male Negro" it was called.[15] Yet many of the men in the Study who lived into the antibiotic era were not the total victims of the Public Health Service (PHS) researchers whose presence in Macon County was fairly episodic. Even Nurse Rivers, who was supposed to monitor the men's activities and keep track of them, only worked part-time on the Study and took other public health, teaching, and school nursing positions. She was not, despite claims otherwise, omnipresent in the men's lives.[16]

The PHS on occasion over the forty years tried to find the men in the Study if they moved around Macon County, or out of the area, using credit bureaus, post office records, and interviews with family members to track them. They were not always successful. Those who moved, and those who could get to doctors in the area, could be treated for other ills (and sometimes even for their syphilis) without the PHS's knowledge or ability to stop it. This the PHS researchers admitted in its articles and correspondence. That they *wanted* the men to remain untreated is certainly true. That they were *not always success-ful* in making this happen is also certainly true, and their own records show it.[17] By the end of the Study the PHS admitted the penicillin some of the men received in haphazard ways, if their ills took them to doctors who either treated them for something else or did not know they were in the Study and treated their syphilis, had primarily defeated it. What factual truth then must we use here?

Central to the horror over the Study is the concept that the PHS stood by as the men passed this sexually transmitted disease on to others they loved. The facts of the Study suggest the men could have passed and did pass the disease on to their wives or other sexual partners both before the Study began and after it was initiated. The subjects were supposed to be chosen because they were in the late latency stage of the disease and therefore no longer contagious. Review of the medical records suggests the PHS was not always so careful in determining this since they relied primarily on the men's memory of when they first noticed syphilitic chancres and lack of visible disease to label them in latency.

A sample of 143 men in the Study showed the men had a median of 19 years after initial infection (beyond contagion at the time), although at least 13 percent of these 143 were in all probability still contagious since they told the PHS they had their first lesions fewer than five years earlier. When the Study ended in 1973, the PHS agreed to treat any wives or children with the disease, *without* determining how they became infected because it was the medically appropriate, morally correct and politically necessary thing to do.[18] Thus 22 wives, 17 children, and 2 grandchildren of men in the Study received lifetime health benefits from the government in the Study's aftermath.[19] Their husbands, fathers and grandfathers may indeed in all likelihood have infected them, but it is also possible they did not.

These numbers receiving lifetime health care as small reparation for the Study add to the confusion, however, over what causes the disease. Sexual transmission during the primary and secondary stages of the disease (up to five years) is the normal method.[20] Despite the determination by the 1920s that syphilis was not a hereditary disease (that is passed down through genes, or more colloquially, through "blood"), but rather a congenital one (that is passed between a still contagious mother to her fetus), family members in Macon County still ask if their own ills of various sorts are caused by the syphilis they might have inherited from their families. Confusing sickle cell trait with a syphilis "trait," I have been asked repeatedly if syphilis, too, is something that can be inherited through a blood tie. Those with children with mental retardation or Down syndrome often use the Study as well to explain their children or grandchildren's health difficulties.[21] All of these factual confusions give power to the Study and fuel its status as a site of memory, a way of seemingly knowing about the African American experience.

JUST THE FICTIONS

The confusions over these facts are then mixed with the fictions that envelop the mythical aspects of the Study. In truth the PHS doctors who ran the Study observed the course of the already acquired and untreated primarily late latent disease in hundreds of African American men in Macon County, Alabama. Yet when the Study is explained it is very often asserted that the doctors went beyond the deception in their planned neglect and *secretly infected or injected* the men with the bacteria that cause syphilis. This virally spread belief is reinforced when photographs of the Study's blood draws circulate, especially when they are cropped to show prominently a black arm and a white hand on a syringe that could, to an unknowing eye, be seen as an injection.

This fictional tale of "infecting" is part of the Study's power legacy. "A rumor," folklorists suggest, "is a 'form of communication though which men [and women] caught together in an ambiguous situation attempt to construct a meaningful interpretation of it by pooling their intellectual resources.'"[22] In a highly racialized and racist country, the idea that white government scientists—believed to be drunk on their power over trusting sharecroppers in need of care—would deliberately and secretly infect black men with a debilitating and sometimes deadly disease seems possible, even if it did not happen here.[23]

This legacy of a belief in deliberate infection often confuses the Study with other horror tales about overzealous and uncaring medical researchers. Those who know about the World War II Nazi and Japanese war experiments link the Study to these horrific deliberate human rights violations. Such a belief also connects the Study to the other major 1960s and 1970s cases of abuse—the injection of cancer cells into elderly patients at the Jewish Chronic Disease Hospital in Brooklyn, New York, and the providing of live hepatitis virus through oral and injecting means to young children with mental retardation at the Willowbrook State School on Staten Island. In addition, to think the men were infected taps deep into our cultural collective consciences' fears of experimentation. It avoids considering the Study's unwitting participants' sexual activities, or those of their parents, since syphilis is primarily, of course, a sexually transmitted disease. To assume the men in the Study were infected, rather than watched for decades, appears to make the racism worse, although it is the very ordinariness of the withholding of treatment and the deceptions necessary to make this possible that ought to frighten us more because this is so normative.[24]

To counter the false claims that the PHS infected the Study's men requires explaining more than that they did not do this. It means understanding something about the biology of syphilis itself. For even if the government doctors had wanted to give the men syphilis, it is a very difficult disease to pass on outside sexual contact, breast-feeding, or congenitally from an infectious mother to her newborn. It demands explaining the doctors could not just inject the spirochetal bacteria that causes syphilis easily from the blood of one person to another, and that centuries of experimentation had demonstrated the difficulties of finding ways experimentally to recreate the disease in the healthy.[25] The *Treponema pallidum*, the spirochete-shaped bacteria that causes syphilis, still to this day cannot be cultured and grown in vitro in a laboratory.

The PHS was involved in studies of direct transfer of the disease, but not in Tuskegee. This required making an inoculum from ground-up infected rabbit testes or from the diseased chancres of individuals that had to be transferred quickly to the next person through scrapings or direct placement in a man's penis. Surely the men in Tuskegee would have remembered and told if this had happened and the extensive records show no shipments of rabbits, lab equipment, or centrifuges to make this possible.[26]

Yet over and over the PHS physicians do become imagined World War II Nazi or Japanese doctors whose racism and power provided by the state allows them to do what we consider dreadful. Or the Study becomes part of an endless litany of abuses of white doctor power on helpless black patients whether it is Dr. J. Marion Sims' 19th-century experiments on slave women with vaginal fistulas or the 20th-century Johns Hopkins studies that involved tracking, but not treating, exposed children in lead-painted apartments.[27] No matter how many truths we tell, the story takes on these multiple fictional qualities because such an assumption is at least possible, if not true.

WHAT IS THE LEGACY?

In the nearly forty years since knowledge of the Study reached the general public, its power has changed. Each year that I teach or lecture on the Study more and more people are shocked that it even occurred, and fewer and fewer have even heard of it. The Study itself, or at least the words "Tuskegee Syphilis Experiment," nevertheless remains available to be used in multiple ways, in part because this knowledge is so sparse and often uninformed, or misinformed. Most recently, for example, groups opposing state funding for stem cell research in Michigan and promoting anti-abortion legislation in Georgia used photographs from the Study in their advertisements directed to African American voters to make the links to the fear of black genocide by a white-dominated government.[28] Details did not matter. Only a few photographs and the words "Tuskegee" need be invoked.

The use of the Study as a site of memory will probably persist regardless of the efforts to get the facts out or to understand why the misremembering happens. These multiple legacies and their usage set the context for the findings of Ralph Katz and his colleagues with their random phone interviews to individuals from differing racial and ethnic groups to ascertain the affect of knowledge of the Study on their stated willingness to participate in clinical trials.[29] Their work questions the orthodoxy that it is knowledge of the Study per se that keeps individuals from minority groups, especially African Americans, from clinical trials that has circulated ever since health educators Stephen Thomas and Sandra Crouse Quinn's article published in 1991 made this argument that was then cited and repeated in historian James H. Jones's second edition of his major book *Bad Blood*.[30] Katz's group's findings suggest it is not something as simple as invoking the Study on an individual level that is its legacy.

Rather the Study's legacy is more collective. The appeal to the words "Tuskegee Syphilis" belongs now to American culture as a site of memory. It is available to be "used and abused," as historians Amy Fairchild and Ronald Bayer argued more than a decade ago.[31] It is made up of facts and fictions and serves as a way to acknowledge fear of medical power, cultural understanding of racism and governmental abuse all at once, or separately if needed, and from the left as well as from the political right. It may not live in the minds of individuals but rather in parts of our collective consciousness. It will, I suspect, remain such a site until justice makes it unnecessary.

THE LEGACY CONTINUES AND CONFOUNDS: AN ADDENDUM TO THE ORIGINAL ESSAY

News events often bring the Tuskegee Syphilis Study back into public view. I never imagined, however, that my own scholarship would make this happen outside an academic venue and to a worldwide audience. As part of the research for my book *Examining Tuskegee*, I went to the archives at the University of Pittsburgh to look at the papers of both Thomas Parran, a former U.S. Surgeon General (1936–48) famous for his concern with syphilis, and John C. Cutler, one of the doctors involved with the Study and a staunch supporter even into the 1990s. What I found in Cutler's papers were reports of an unpublished PHS project in Guatemala from 1946–48 that involved the actual inoculation of prostitutes, prisoners, mental patients, and soldiers with syphilis and then their treatment (although not all) with penicillin. I left the story out of my book because the details were too complicated, presented it a professional meeting in May 2010, and then wrote it up for a policy history journal to be published in January 2011.[32] To make sure I had the medical details and PHS culture correct, I shared the pre-publication paper with Dr. David Sencer, the former director of the Centers for Disease Control, whom I had met in the course of my research.

Sencer, shocked and concerned by my findings, asked if he could show the paper to officials at the CDC. Deeply troubled by my article, their response was to send their leading syphilologist, Dr. John Douglas, to the Pittsburgh archives and to send his report (which supported my findings and detailed the medical consequences) and my paper up the chain of the command, where it eventually ended up in the White House.[33] On October 1, 2010, there was a formal dual apology from both the Secretaries of State and Health and Human Services, a phone call from President Obama to President Colon in Guatemala, and Obama requesting his Bioethics Commission to explore current human subject protections.

The media coverage of this unprecedented American apology for a study that was done six decades ago became worldwide, and I fielded questions from the *New York Times* to Chinese national television as thousands of stories on this were filed. Once again, in part because of my role as a historian of the Syphilis Study in Tuskegee, the question of inoculation came up. Once again, I had to explain over and over the differences between the two studies: the men in Tuskegee were never infected by the government nor were effective treatment attempts made; the men and women in Guatemala were given the disease by the government and effective treatment efforts were part of the research. A future historian will have to determine whether the exposure of the story of the inoculation studies in Guatemala has now undone all the efforts to explain what really happened in Tuskegee and what effects on the "legacy" this new site of memory will create.

Susan M. Reverby, PhD (McLean Professor in the History of Ideas and Professor of Women's and Gender Studies, Wellesley College), is a historian of American women, nursing, race and health care. Her books include her edited Tuskegee's Truths: Rethinking the Tuskegee Syphilis Study *(2000) and her prize-winning* Examining Tuskegee: The Infamous Syphilis Study and its Legacy *(2009). She was a member of the Legacy Committee that organized for a federal apology for the study. Her most recent article on the PHS's inoculation STD studies in Guatemala led to worldwide media attention and another apology from the White House.*

NOTES

1. Susan M. Reverby, ed. *Tuskegee's Truths: Rethinking the Tuskegee Syphilis Study* (Chapel Hill: University of North Carolina Press, 2000); Susan M. Reverby, *Examining*

Tuskegee: The Infamous Syphilis Study and its Legacy (Chapel Hill: University of North Carolina Press, 2009).

2. Robert O'Meally and Geneviève Fabre, "Introduction," in *History and Memory in African-American Culture*, ed. Geneviève Fabre and Robert O'Meally (New York: Oxford University Press, 1994), p. 7.

3. Ibid., p. 6.

4. "Trust Your Doctor," *Saturday Night Live*, aired on NBC on October 26, 2007.

5. Barclay quoted in Karen Fields, "What One Cannot Remember Mistakenly," in Fabre and O'Meally, ed. *History and Memory*, p. 154; Stephen Colbert, "The Word," October 17, 2005, *The Colbert Report*, Comedy Central, http://www.colbertnation .com/the-colbert-report-videos/24039/october-17-2005/the-word---truthiness, accessed June 4, 2010.

6. It is impossible to capture in a quantitative manner how often factual mistakes about the Study are made, even as they appear daily in whispers, websites, scholarly treatises, and evening newscasts. Even a "Google alert" or a continual LexisNexis search for "Tuskegee Syphilis" cannot collect all the sites of knowledge production about the Study. There are, however, a series of common beliefs that reappear over and over. For an earlier discussion of fact and fiction, see Susan M. Reverby, "More than Fact and Fiction: Cultural Memory and the Tuskegee Syphilis Study," *Hastings Center Report* 31 (September–October 2001): 22–28.

7. There is no evidence that there are shared beliefs in *a* nonexistent singular black community, see Dennis Medina, "Intelligent Action: An Interview with Adolph Reed," CUNY Graduate Center Advocate, May 26, 2010, http://www.gcadvocate.com/2010/05 /intelligent-action-an-interview-with-adolph-reed/, accessed May 27, 2010.

8. ABC aired a *Primetime Live* segment on the Study in 1992 and HBO aired "Deadly Deception," an hour-long documentary in 1993. For more on the post-1972 life of the Study, see Reverby, *Examining Tuskegee*.

9. There is an enormous historical literature on historical memory and American identity. See, for example, Marita Sturken, *Tangled Memories* (Berkeley: University of California Press, 1997) and David Blight, *Race and Reunion* (Cambridge: Harvard University Press, 2001).

10. Historians have long bemoaned the public's fascination with the good story rather than the historian's search for meaning and facts. See Tom Bartlett, "Why isn't History More Interesting?" *The Chronicle of Higher Education*, April 16, 2010, http:// chronicle.com/blogPost/Why-Isnt-History-More-Inte/231533/, accessed April 17, 2010; Peter N. Stearns, *Meaning over Memory: Recasting the Teaching of History and Culture* (Chapel Hill: University of North Carolina Press, 1993).

11. Wikipedia's openness adds to the problem. Last year I discovered that a strange name had been added as one of the PHS physicians in the Tuskegee Syphilis Study entry. I tracked the name down to a high school actor in New York and assumed it might have been some joke by his friends. I corrected the entry on Wikipedia. However, by then two African American–oriented websites had repeated the Wikipedia entry with the false name. I tried to correct these but found it difficult to contact the owners of the sites. Meanwhile, I was told by someone working on a history of the

Study that this name was relevant even though it was clearly false. The existence of the web makes the life of false information seemingly endless.

12. These are the numbers first reported by Jean Heller in the 1972 Associated Press story that made the Study public, "Syphilis Victims in U.S. Study Were Untreated for 40 Years," *New York Times,* July 26, 1972 and reprinted in Reverby, *Tuskegee's Truths,* pp. 116–118. James H. Jones uses these numbers in *Bad Blood* (New York: Free Press, 1981, second edition, 1993).

13. Patricia Smith, "Praise be these old Black Men," *Boston Globe,* May 23, 1997, http://www.english.illinois.edu/maps/poets/s_z/p_smith/columns.htm, accessed June 9, 2010.

14. See longer discussion in Reverby, *Examining Tuskegee,* pp. 111–134.

15. For a list of the articles published on the Study before 1973, see Reverby, *Tuskegee's Truths,* pp. 606–607.

16. Rivers is the subject of multiple interpretations. See Reverby, ed., *Tuskegee's Truths,* pp. 321–398, 527–554; Reverby, *Examining Tuskegee,* pp. 167–186.

17. Reverby, *Examining Tuskegee,* pp. 111–134.

18. Ibid., p. 117.

19. Carol Kaesuk Yoon, "Families Emerge as Silent Victims of Tuskegee Syphilis Experiments," *New York Times,* May 12, 1997, pp. A1, A 12 and reprinted in Reverby, ed. *Tuskegee's Truths,* pp. 457–460.

20. Women sexual partners/wives of the men could have then passed the disease on to their children if they were still infectious at the time of birth.

21. I have been speaking with family members of the Study in Macon County since the mid 1990s. This always comes up as a question.

22. Sociologist Tamotsu Shibutani, quoted in Patricia Turner and Gary Alan Fine, *Whispers on the Color Line: Rumor and Race in America* (Berkeley: University of California Press, 2004), pp. 58–59.

23. For an example of when infecting did occur, see Susan M. Reverby, "'Normal Exposure' and Inoculation Syphilis: A PHS 'Tuskegee' Doctor in Guatemala," 1946–48," *Journal of Policy History* 23 (Winter 2011): 1–23.

24. Reverby, "More than Fact and Fiction."

25. Joan Sherwood, "Syphilization: Human Experimentation in the Search for a Syphilis Vaccine in the Nineteenth Century," *Journal of the History of Medicine* 54 (July 1999): 364–386 and Susan E. Lederer, *Subjected to Science* (Baltimore: Johns Hopkins University Press, 1995).

26. Reverby, "'Normal Exposure;'" Harold J. Magnuson et al., "Inoculation Syphilis in Human Volunteers," *Medicine* 35 (February 1956): 33–82; John C. Cutler, "An Experimental Resurvey of the Basic Factors Concerned in Prophylaxis in Syphilis," Unpublished typescript, Box 1, Folder 9, Cutler Papers, University Archives, University of Pittsburgh, Pittsburgh, PA.

27. Vanessa Northington Gamble, "Under the Shadow of Tuskegee: African Americans and Health Care," *American Journal of Public Health* 87 (November 1997): 1773–87 and reprinted in Reverby, ed. *Tuskegee's Truths,* pp. 431–442. This view of the unending stream of use of black patients is made most forcefully in Harriet

Washington, *Medical Apartheid* (New York: Doubleday, 2007). See Susan M. Reverby, "Inclusion and Exclusion: The Politics of History, Difference and Medical Research," *Journal of the History of Medicine* 63 (January 2008): 103–113.

28. "The Truth about Stem Cell Science," University of Michigan Health System Newsroom, October 27, 2008, http://www2.med.umich.edu/prmc/media/newsroom /details.cfm?ID=800, accessed June 7, 2010; Kathryn Joyce, "Abortion as 'Black Genocide': An Old Scare Tactic Re-Emerges," *The Public Eye-Political Research Associates,"* April 29, 2010, http://www.publiceye.org/magazine/v25n1/abortion-black-genocide .html, accessed June 7, 2010.

29. See TLP Study articles by RV Katz et al. in Appendix IV.

30. Stephen B. Thomas and Sandra Crouse Quinn, "The Tuskegee Syphilis Study, 1932–1972, Implications for HIV Education and AIDS Risk Education Programs in the Black Community," *American Journal of Public Health* 81 (1991): 1448–1505 and reprinted in Reverby, ed. *Tuskegee's Truths*, pp. 404–417; Jones, *Bad Blood*.

31. "Uses and Abuses of Tuskegee," *Science* 284 (7 March 1999): 919–21, reprinted in Reverby, ed. *Tuskegee's Truths*, pp. 589–603.

32. See footnote 24.

33. The government's response and Douglas' report are available at http://www .hhs.gov/1946inoculationstudy/, accessed 30 December 2010.

Essay 4

Tuskegee Legacy

The Role of the Social Determinants of Health

David Satcher

In the mid-1990s as director of the Centers for Disease Control and Prevention (CDC), I had the opportunity to appoint a national committee to revisit the Tuskegee Syphilis Study and to make recommendations for national consideration. The committee's report was presented to President Clinton and resulted in a Presidential Apology for the Tuskegee Syphilis Study which had lasted for forty years.

Approximately 10 years later, I served as a member of the World Health Organization's (WHO) Commission on Social Determinants of Health (CSDH). The commission's report,[1] released in London in November, 2008, was released in Geneva by the WHO in January 2009.

The purpose of this essay is to examine, in retrospect, the role of social determinants of health (SDH) in the Tuskegee Study. Social determinants of health have been defined as the conditions in which people are born, grow, learn, work, age, and die, and the impact that those conditions have on health outcomes. These conditions include employment or work, education, environment, poverty, urban and rural settings, and social exclusion, to name a few. It is from that perspective that I reexamine the Tuskegee Syphilis Study.

THE TUSKEGEE STUDY OF UNTREATED SYPHILIS IN THE NEGRO MALE

In 1932 Tuskegee Institute in conjunction with the United States Public Health Service (USPHS) initiated a study of 399 men with syphilis and a

41

control group of 201 men without, in order to observe the natural history or progression of the disease. The men were neither told that they had syphilis, nor were they given appropriate treatment for the condition. In fact, they were told that they had "bad blood," a familiar term for a variety of disorders, and were given free medical examinations, free meals, and burial insurance for participating in the study. As treatment modalities advanced to the proven effectiveness of penicillin in 1947, these men were still denied the treatment.

THE ROLE OF SOCIAL DETERMINANTS OF HEALTH

The study subjects have generally been described as poor, illiterate sharecroppers who had limited access to adequate health care. They were born, lived, and worked in the rural South. All of these descriptors are social determinants of health, conditions that had a direct impact on their attitudes, daily lives, and health outcomes. According to a Tuskegee University report,[2] "The men were offered what most Negroes could only dream of in terms of medical care and survivors' insurance. The men were enticed and enrolled in the study with incentives including: medical exams, rides to and from the clinics, meals on examination days, free treatment for minor ailments and guarantees that provisions would be made after their deaths in terms of burial stipends paid to their survivors."

What the men did not know was that their primary usefulness to the study would be the information obtained from their bodies, via autopsies, after they were dead. Certainly, the conditions into which they were born, lived, and worked had a major impact upon their health and their condition at death. These men and their families suffered needlessly for years because they were taken advantage of in what has been called one of the worst biomedical research studies ever undertaken in this country. The Tuskegee Syphilis Study poignantly demonstrates the role that SDH play in our lives.

THE CDC CONNECTION

I learned about the Tuskegee Syphilis Study in 1972, 40 years after its inception, first from an article in the *New York Times* condemning the study, and then from the writings of Dr. James Jones, a historian who wrote the book, *Bad Blood: The Tuskegee Syphilis Experiment.* The ending of the study in 1972 was also the beginning of a thorough assessment of what had happened— when, how, and why?

As of 1959 the responsibility for the study was under the auspices of the Centers for Disease Control and Prevention (CDC)—an agency for which I would serve as director, from 1993 to 1998. During my tenure as director, an outstanding committee, The Tuskegee Syphilis Study Legacy Committee, was appointed to examine the "Tuskegee Legacy" and make recommendations for how the history should be used in developing policies and programs going forward. The committee was chaired by the physician and anthropologist Dr. Vanessa Northington Gamble.

A major recommendation in the 1997 Tuskegee Syphilis Study Legacy Committee Report[3] was to seek a Presidential Apology to help draw attention to the study and its implications and to speak to the suffering of survivors and their families. The committee made very clear the importance of an apology which not only looked at this willful experience in American history and in the lives of individuals and families, but it also felt the apology should point to a future where the risk of this kind of experiment ever occurring again in America would be minimal.

My responsibility was to present the committee's report to President Clinton and to convince him to issue an apology with the associated goals for the future. I made a special trip to Washington to meet with my immediate boss, Donna Shalala, the Secretary of the Department of Health and Human Services. We met at the end of the day and our discussion went well into the evening. Donna Shalala was so moved by the report that she felt we should contact President Clinton as soon as possible. With some effort we were able to speak with him that evening. As usual, he was a quick study and seemingly understood the significance of this request right away. He also agreed that it was important—that he owed not only an apology which regretted the past, but one that included a plan for a better future.

THE PRESIDENT'S APOLOGY

Over the next few months, we worked with colleagues within the Department of Health and Human Services (HHS), the leadership of the survivor group from Tuskegee and their attorney, and the leadership of Tuskegee University to plan for the apology. On March 16, 1997, President Clinton delivered the apology,[4] saying what the government had done was "deeply, profoundly and morally wrong. It was an outrage to our commitment to integrity and equality for all our citizens." Additionally:

> To the survivors, to the wives and family members, the children and the grandchildren, I say what you know: No power on Earth can give you back the lives lost, the pain suffered, the years of internal torment and anguish. What was done cannot be undone. But we can end the silence. We can stop turning our heads away. We can look at you in the eye and finally say, on

behalf of the American people: what the United States government did was shameful, and I am sorry.

I think it is important to examine the five goals set forth in the president's apology, for a different future in medicine and public health, in light of the Tuskegee Syphilis Study. First, the United States government would help to build a lasting memorial to the Tuskegee Syphilis Study participants, at Tuskegee University. This would be a center for bioethics and research in health care. It would also serve as a museum of the study, support efforts to address its legacy, and strengthen bioethics training. Two, a commitment to increase community involvement with public health to begin restoring lost trust. The secretary was ordered to present a plan within six months for better engaging communities, especially minority communities, in research and health care. Three, a commitment to strengthen researchers' training in bioethics, not only at the Tuskegee Bioethics Center but also in programs throughout the country. Four, to develop and provide a post-graduate fellowship to train bioethicists especially among African Americans and other minority groups. Five, President Clinton extended the charter of the National Bioethics Advisory Commission, which was due to expire in 1997, to October 1999.

Today the National Center for Bioethics in Research and Health Care, established in 1999, is still in operation. Last year I had the opportunity to speak at its 10th anniversary and was presented the Sankofa Bird Award in Ethics. However, the sustainability of the center is still in question in that it was never endowed. Research in medicine and public health, as well as researchers in medicine and public health, and those who care for patients are required on a biannual basis to demonstrate an understanding of policies and practices governing patient care and safety and confidentiality. There are also guidelines regulating requirements for representation of community participation and research funded by the National Institutes of Health (NIH) and other Federal agencies. There are also fellowships in bioethics funded both publicly and privately at universities throughout the nation, and finally, the term of the National Bioethics Advisory Commission was indeed extended.

FURTHER ANALYSIS OF THE IMPORTANCE OF SOCIAL DETERMINANTS OF HEALTH

The issues of SDH and how they played out in the decision to carry out the study, and the ability of the USPHS to maintain the involvement of 399 African American men without treatment for 40 years, has not been adequately addressed by our government. This neglect may impact our future risk for studies similar to the Tuskegee Syphilis Study.

In 1932 and during most of the Tuskegee Syphilis Study, the social conditions that were dominant were those that characterized much of the American history of race relations. Poverty, social exclusion, ignorance, and little or no access to health care describe the plight of African Americans in Tuskegee and much of America, but especially in the South and especially in Alabama, my home state.

Discrimination in education, employment, income, access to health care, and violence and threats of violence prevailed in the plight of the Negro in the South and again especially in Alabama. I, too, observed African American men working in the foundries of Anniston, Alabama, who were unable to apply for certain jobs because of their race. It was understood that certain jobs were reserved for white men only. And so the system in place was meant to prevent African American men from advancing beyond a certain point in much of the work that existed throughout the South. And certainly that was true in Tuskegee—that African American men would agree to participate in a study in which they thought they were being treated for syphilis is quite understandable given the nature of race relations, discrimination, education, communication, and wealth in the life and experience of African Americans in the South in 1932 and during the subsequent 40-year period of this study.

The underrepresentation of African Americans in the health professions, which continues today, was even worse during the period 1932–1972. Also, African American physicians were excluded from most of the hospitals in the South, until the Hill-Burden Act of the mid-1960s. This meant that African American physicians in the care of their patients had very limited access to hospitals and most of their patients suffered and died at home. A story which I have told many times is about my near bout with death from whooping cough and pneumonia at the age of two. An African American physician, Dr. Jackson, came out to our home to see me, and even though he projected that I would not live out the week, he was not able to put me in the hospital. That was how it was for most African American families and African American children during that time.

RECOMMENDATIONS OF THE COMMISSION ON SOCIAL DETERMINANTS OF HEALTH

In January 2009 WHO released the report of the CSDH, a commission on which I served from 2005–2008. The commission was established by the WHO director, General J. W. Lee, to help get at the root of health inequity globally and to start a grassroots movement toward health equity. Inequities in health occur within countries, as with disparities in health in this country, and between countries, and often relate directly to factors such as income, education, and social cohesion. Our task was to study the impact of SDH by visiting several countries that were visibly affected and countries that had targeted SDH as a way of moving toward health equity. Thus, the goal of the commission was to define a strategy for achieving global health equity with a focus on SDH. The commission found that the distribution of power and resources were paramount in influencing health outcomes and that they must be more equally distributed in order to achieve global health equity.

The commission recommended that the issue of health inequity needed to be attacked at the highest levels of government—locally, state, and nationally. It also recommended that when policies are made in areas of social determinants, that the health impact of these policies be addressed and considered. Thus, with new programs, policies, and environmental controls, zoning, employment, education, and social interventions, there should be a requirement to access and report the potential health impact.

CONCLUSION

It is true that syphilis was and is more common among African Americans than the majority population in America. This is also true of HIV/AIDS and why we should never stop appealing to individual responsibility in terms of lifestyle. We must also elevate our attack on the social conditions, especially poverty, discrimination, ignorance, disparities in health and disparities in access to quality health care which we see in all of these areas. Perhaps no cases or examples better illustrate the critical role of social determinants of health than the Tuskegee Syphilis Study. While this was not a topic for discussion in President Clinton's apology, it must be an issue as we move forward, if we are ever to achieve the goals set forth in the Tuskegee Apology and prevent similar travesties from happening.

So there was a Tuskegee Syphilis Study that ended disgracefully. There was a Presidential Apology, which some of the participants of the study and their families participated in, and there were policies and programs put in place in effect to preserve the legacy of the Tuskegee Syphilis Study, to make biomedical research more ethical, and to assure that this could never happen again.

David Satcher, MD, PhD, director of The Satcher Health Leadership Institute and The Center for Excellence on Health Disparities, established in 2006 at the Morehouse School of Medicine in Atlanta, Georgia, was sworn in as the 16th Surgeon General of the United States in 1998. His tenure of public service includes serving as director of the Centers for Disease Control and Prevention (CDC). He was the first person to have served as director of the CDC and then surgeon general of the United States. Dr. Satcher has also held top leadership positions at the Charles R. Drew University for Medicine and Science and the Meharry Medical College.

NOTES

1. CSDH (2008). *Closing the gap in a generation: health equity through action on the social determinants of health. Final Report of the Commission on Social Determinants of Health.* Geneva, World Health Organization.

2. *Information About the USPHS Syphilis Study.* All content Copyright 2003—2010 Tuskegee University and WorldNow. Available at: http://www.tuskegee.edu/Global /story.asp?S=6377076. Accessed July 26, 2010.

3. Final Report of the Tuskegee Syphilis Study Legacy Committee—May 20, 1996. Available at: http://www.hsl.virginia.edu/historical/medical_history/bad_blood/report .cfm. Accessed July 26, 2010.

4. Apology for Study Done in Tuskegee. The White House Office of the Press secretary. Remarks by the President in Apology for Study Done in Tuskegee. Available at: http://clinton4.nara.gov/textonly/New/Remarks/Fri/19970516-898.html. Accessed July 8, 2010.

Essay 5

Toward the Ethical Conduct of Science and a Socially Just World

Mary E. Northridge

Reflecting on the infamous US Public Health Service Syphilis Study at Tuskegee (Study) is a sobering assignment. One is forced to confront the tragic American history of racism that pre-dated the Study, morphed during it, and lives on in altered forms.[1] The prism through which this essay confronts the Study and analyzes its legacy is the scientific and scholarly papers chronicled in the *American Journal of Public Health* (*Journal*), now in its hundredth year of publication. Given the century-long time frame and the breadth of topics covered by the *Journal*, this case study approach may prove insightful in the context of the other essays in this volume, as the public health science that is funded, conducted, and published assuredly mirrors societal values.

This choice of prism further recognizes what former Editor-in-Chief of the *Journal* Alfred Yankauer acknowledged as the forty-year silence of the medical, public health, and social science journals in condemning the Study.[2] He questioned readers, "Does the silence tell us something about our own buried biases and stereotypes that operate, often without our conscious knowledge, to influence ourselves and our conscious behavior?"[2] (p. 1406)

Finally, among the seven key papers published on the Tuskegee Legacy Project that serve as the foundation for the essays in this current collective book [see Appendix B] is one that originally appeared in the *Journal* titled, "Awareness of the Tuskegee Syphilis Study and the US presidential apology and their influence on minority participation in biomedical research."[3] Findings were that blacks were nearly four times as likely as whites to have heard of the Study, more than twice as likely to have correctly named

49

Clinton as the president who made the apology, and two to three times more likely to have been willing to participate in biomedical studies despite having heard about the Study or the Presidential Apology. The authors concluded that, "These marked differences likely reflect the cultural reality in the black community, which has been accustomed to increased risks in many activities."[3] (p. 1137) And so, the question posed in this reflective essay is, "Has the legacy of Tuskegee moved us toward the ethical conduct of science and a more socially just world?"

BLATANT RACISM AND SCIENTIFIC ARROGANCE

Historian Vanessa Gamble cogently argued that, "The Tuskegee Syphilis Study has emerged as the most prominent example of medical racism because it confirms, if not authenticates, long-held and deeply entrenched beliefs within the black community."[4] (p. 1775) Undeniably, in the pages of the *Journal* at the time the Study was initiated, the blatant racism is palpable at multiple levels. The article, "Control of syphilis in a Southern rural area: a preliminary report"[5] by L. E. Burney published in the *Journal* in 1939 serves to illustrate the point. The stated purpose of the instituted program was "to determine the most effective method of controlling syphilis in the southern rural Negro."[5] (p. 1006) Burney despaired that learning the source of infection was practically impossible. "Naturally, as promiscuous as these people are, it is impossible to obtain the source of infection obtained 2, 4, or 10 years ago."[5] (p. 1009) He also commended the use of force by the mayor of one small town to ensure patients received treatment. "We gave him the names of a few incorrigible ringleaders. He sentenced them to jail or the clinic. They chose the clinic. This has had a beneficial effect upon the other patients in this community."[5] (p. 1009) Finally, he empathized with the only two physicians in the three counties of interest who verbally objected to the program. "They feel that these Negroes, whose average wage is but $6 a week, can afford to pay them $2 to $3 a week for anti-syphilitic treatment. Their criticism is sincere and frank, and we try to cooperate with them whenever possible."[5] (p. 1011)

It was also disconcerting to read a 1954 report published in the *Journal*—seven years after penicillin was accepted as the treatment of choice for syphilis in 1947—that cited the then 20-year study of untreated syphilis by the Division of Venereal Disease at Tuskegee, Ala.[6] "Our findings in the Tuskegee study show that untreated syphilis reduces life expectancy by 17 per cent."[6] (p. 357) The tone of the racism had changed, but still there was no protest from the *Journal* or its readers that Study participants with syphilis remained untreated with penicillin.[2] Instead, as late as 1965 and after 30 years of follow-up of the Tuskegee participants, the Study investigators took pains in the *Journal* to defend the serological tests for syphilis that were performed,[7] and expressed umbrage at the word "trick" being used in a brief *Journal* bibliography that recommended securing agreement among viewers in reading the tests.[8] The emphasis was decidedly on upholding the scientific standards of the Study rather than protecting the health and lives of the participants.

ETHICAL DEBATE AND ENDORSED PRINCIPLES

After 40 years, a story by the Associated Press led to a public outcry and ultimately the official end of the Study in 1972. Belatedly, an ethical debate ensued in the *Journal*. The Study was invoked to, for example, protect "captive" populations such as those in prisons and institutions.[9] Monitoring of ongoing research was recommended as it "would help to avoid a repetition of experiences of the Tuskegee Study, where penicillin was withheld from the subjects long after it became the accepted cure for syphilis."[9] (p. 547) Finally, the American Public Health Association urged the Department of Health, Education, and Welfare to review its policies and to adopt the following principles:

1. Biomedical research will be conducted upon members of a captive population only if the research design is such that a captive population is the only population which will allow for the satisfaction of the research objectives. The decision of necessity of captive population will be made by the Committee on Human Subjects Research of the proposed institution, and not by the investigator.
2. Committees on Human Subject Research in institutional settings will follow the most current guidelines by the Food and Drug Administration and/or the Department of Health, Education, and Welfare relating to this question, and will be composed, in addition to the required membership, of representatives of the proposed subject population, and non–institutionally affiliated professionals selected by the subjects and other appropriate citizens from the community at large.
3. The question of informed consent should be followed to the letter and will be strengthened by including the principles listed below:

   a. Prospective participants should be informed of the sources of funding of the experiment and of the purposes to which the results of the experimentation will be put (to the extent these are known at the time).
   b. Participants should be informed of the existence of the Committee on Human Subjects Research and invited to communicate with

    it regarding any concerns arising out of their involvement in the experiment.

  c. Participants should be informed concerning changed circumstances, including heretofore unknown side effects or cures for their particular ailments.[9] (p. 547)

From that point on, the *Journal* became an academic vehicle for ethical debate on the pressing public health priorities of the times, with certain authors invoking the Study and others questioning its aptness. For instance, in their historical paper, "The Tuskegee Syphilis Study, 1932 to 1972: implications for HIV education and AIDS risk education programs in the black community," Stephen Thomas and Sandra Crouse Quinn argued for an open and honest discussion of the Study to facilitate the process of rebuilding trust between the black community and public health authorities.[10] In their words: "The AIDS epidemic has exposed the Tuskegee Syphilis Study as a historical marker for the legitimate discontent of blacks with the public health system. In the absence of a cure for AIDS, education remains our best chance to stop the spread of HIV infection. We must discuss the feeling within the black community that AIDS is a form of genocide, a feeling justified by the history of the Tuskegee study."[10] (p. 1504)

    Gershon Grunfeld instead stressed the dissimilarities between the Tuskegee Syphilis Study and HIV/AIDS programs.[11] He outlined important differences in protocols, supervision by independent review boards, informed consent, and prevention of subjects from obtaining known effective treatments, and emphasized the safeguards then in place to "prevent studies similar to the one conducted in Tuskegee."[11] (p. 1176) Don Des Jarlais and Bruce Stepherson identified one specific detail of the Study that had disturbing implications for AIDS prevention: "[T]he research for the Tuskegee study was initiated in the absence of adequate funding to provide needed treatment. We have not solved our racial problems with respect to public health policy and practice in the United States, and we may be about to repeat mistakes generated (at least in part) by a lack of funding for what should be considered public health necessities."[12] (p. 1393)

    This tension between adequate resources and egalitarian justice continued to play out in the *Journal* by invoking the transgressions of the Study through, for example, critiques of maternal-fetal HIV transmission prevention trials in developing nations[13,14] and the Kennedy Krieger Institute Lead Paint Study in Baltimore.[15–17] With regard to the conduct of trials in developing nations, George Annas and Michael Grodin contended that, "Actual delivery of health care requires more than just paying lip service to the principles of the Universal Declaration of Human Rights; it requires a real commitment to human rights and a willingness on the part of the developed countries to take economic, social, and cultural rights as seriously as political and civil rights."[13] (p. 562) Meanwhile, Ronald Bayer countered, "The tragedy of the recent trials is that they bear a profound moral taint, not of a malevolent research design but, rather, of a world economic order that makes effective prophylaxis for the interruption of maternal-fetal HIV transmission available but unaffordable for many—this is true, as well, for a host of treatments for AIDS and other diseases."[14] (p. 570) With regard to the *Grimes v Kennedy Krieger Institute, Inc.* legal case, Anna C. Mastroianni and Jeffrey Kahn reasoned, "Public trust may be the key, since without it there can be no research—no subjects for research projects, and no funding to support them."[16] (p. 1076) David Buchanan and Franklin Miller later warned that "Dogmatic stances that preclude research aimed at evaluating cost-effective interventions on grounds of egalitarian justice will result in research paralysis and policy stagnation, thus guaranteeing the continuing neglect of the needs of disadvantaged populations."[17] (p. 786)

In 2002, recognizing societal demand for explicit attention to ethics arising from "technological advances that create new possibilities and, with them, new ethical dilemmas; new challenges to health, such as the advent of HIV; and abuses of power, such as the Tuskegee study of syphilis"[18] (p. 1057) the *Journal* published the following Principles of the Ethical Practice of Public Health:

1. Public health should address principally the fundamental causes of disease and requirements for health, aiming to prevent adverse health outcomes.
2. Public health should achieve community health in a way that respects the rights of individuals in the community.
3. Public health policies, programs, and priorities should be developed and evaluated through processes that ensure an opportunity for input from community members.
4. Public health should advocate for, or work for the empowerment of, disenfranchised community members, ensuring that the basic resources and conditions necessary for health are accessible to all people in the community.
5. Public health should seek the information needed to implement effective policies and programs that protect and promote health.
6. Public health institutions should provide communities with the information they have that is needed for decisions on policies or programs and should obtain the community's consent for their implementation.
7. Public health institutions should act in a timely manner on the information they have within the resources and the mandate given to them by the public.

8. Public health programs and policies should incorporate a variety of approaches that anticipate and respect diverse values, beliefs, and cultures in the community.
9. Public health programs and policies should be implemented in a manner that most enhances the physical and social environment.
10. Public health institutions should protect the confidentiality of information that can bring harm to an individual or community if made public. Exceptions must be justified on the basis of the high likelihood of significant harm to the individual or others.
11. Public health institutions should ensure the professional competence of their employees.
12. Public health institutions and their employees should engage in collaborations and affiliations in ways that build the public's trust and the institution's effectiveness.[18] (p. 1058)

In its posted Instructions for Authors, the *Journal* affirms that it adheres to these principles, and all prospective authors are required to state whether or not they have complied with this code upon official submission of their papers.

HEALTH DISPARITIES AND COMMUNITY ENGAGEMENT

In the present era, the *Journal* overtly endorses public health research, policy, practice, and education papers on eliminating health disparities among population groups and engaging communities in the research enterprise. In both of these broad-based endeavors, the legacy of Tuskegee is clearly manifest. In a paper published in the landmark February 2003 issue of the *Journal* devoted to Racism and Health, Nancy Krieger castigated "the flawed research agenda egregiously exemplified by the Tuskegee syphilis study, unnaturally intended to determine whether the 'natural history' of untreated syphilis in blacks was the same as that previously observed in whites, in light of hypothesized differences in their nervous systems."[18] (p. 195)

With regard to the structural barriers to participation of older adults in clinical trials, Angelica Herrera and colleagues conjectured, "The unethical treatment of African Americans in research, epitomized by the Tuskegee Syphilis Study, may partly explain why older ethnic minorities may be reluctant to participate in today's clinical trials, despite achievements in human participant protections."[19] (p. S105) Meanwhile, Donald Musa and colleagues examined trust in the health care system and use of preventive health services by older black and white adults.[20] According to the authors, there were "no significant racial differences in trust in health information from the local health department and the Centers for Disease Control and Prevention, which we found surprising, given widespread knowledge of the Tuskegee Syphilis Study (conducted by the US Public Health Service) and the broader history of racial discrimination in the US health care system. However, blacks reported significantly more trust than did whites in health information sources like family, friends, and church or religious leaders, reflecting the importance of informal social networks, faith communities, and extended family for blacks."[20] (p. 1297)

There has also been ongoing debate in the *Journal* about how to ethically engage communities in public health research given the public outrage and policy response to the Tuskegee Syphilis Study. By all accounts, the process employed is crucial if not yet perfected. Sandra Crouse Quinn posited that Community Advisory Boards offer "an opportunity to adopt a relationships paradigm that enables researchers to anticipate and address the context in which communities understand risks and benefits, and individuals give consent."[21] (p. 918) She thus advised conducting research to understand the role of Community Advisory Boards in the informed consent process.[21] Another strategy was proposed by Moriah McSharry McGrath and colleagues who conducted comparative case studies of three research organizations at a single medical center.[22] They concluded that Institutional Review Boards have "the authority and the moral imperative to act against the productivity pressures of the research system and for the good of research participants and their communities."[22] (p. 1513) Finally, Beverly Xaviera Watkins and colleagues recommended a Community Ethical Review Board model with periodic communication between the Community Advisory Board and the Institutional Review Board to fulfill the increased obligation to protect the rights and welfare of human participants when some or all of them are economically or educationally disadvantaged.[23]

REFLECTION

In reviewing the papers published in the *Journal* over the past 100 years, it is indeed likely that the legacy of the Tuskegee Syphilis Study has moved us toward the ethical conduct of science. Nonetheless, processes for improved community engagement and rigorous, balanced, and transparent ethical review remain paramount, as does the importance of maintaining "clear and unwavering respect for the dignity and worth of individuals across racial, gender, religious, sexual, tribal, ethnic, and geographic lines."[24] (p. 1707) In the view of Barry Bozeman and colleagues: "Tuskegee surely motivated the complex regulatory system for research involving human participants from vulnerable groups and it continues to fuel public and regulatory scrutiny of research institutions. However, no amount of outrage or intolerance for historically unethical science behavior is enough to overcome contemporary institutional organizational inadequacies and, therefore, it should be no surprise that exploitation of vulnerable populations still occurs."[25] (p. 1550) Community-based participatory research and other group processes in general are subject to improvement by observation, evaluation, and planned change, even as effective institutions and processes remain vulnerable to those who work within them. Thus, it is critical to remember that people are people, and researchers ought never become too detached from their research participants.[25]

Tragically, however, the legacy of the Tuskegee Syphilis Study has failed to move us toward a socially just world. While the overt racism that led to the flawed science of the Study is no longer apparent in the *Journal*, documented health disparities between those with power and resources and those without continue unabated. The view expressed by Steven Whitman in 1974—right after the Study was officially halted—rings just as true nearly 40 years later: "Yes, it hurts to see the tabulations of white versus black health levels. Yes, it gives overt racists a chance to say loudly what is in the minds and hearts of many liberals. But these are not reasons to stop. Rather, they are reasons to continue on, to intensify the pain so that the disease, and not only its symptoms, is purged."[26] (p. 172) It is the struggle for health equity that the *Journal* now participates in fully until the just world so desperately sought becomes the lived reality for everyone.

Mary E. Northridge, PhD, MPH, is editor-in-chief of the American Journal of Public Health *and was professor of clinical sociomedical sciences (in dental medicine) at the Columbia University Mailman School of Public Health at the time of this research and writing, where she still holds a part-time appointment. She is currently in the Department of Epidemiology and Health Promotion at the NYU College of Dentistry. Professor Northridge has enduring interests in social and environmental determinants of health, including oral health, and an emerging focus in the utility of systems science to integrate and sustain holistic health and health care for older adults.*

NOTES

1. Northridge M. E. Claiming Tuskegee. Book review of *Examining Tuskegee: The Infamous Tuskegee Study and Its Legacy* by Susan M. Reverby. *Health Aff.* 2010, 29(6):1271–1271.

2. Yankauer, A. The neglected lesson of the Tuskegee study. *Am J Public Health.* 1998;88(9):1406.

3. Katz, R. V., Kegeles, S. S., Kressin, N. R., Green, B. L., James, S. A., Wang, M. Q., Russell, S. L., and Claudio C. Awareness of the Tuskegee Syphilis Study and the US presidential apology and their influence on minority participation in biomedical research. *Am J Public Health.* 2008, 98(6):1137–1142.

4. Gamble, V. N. Under the shadow of Tuskegee: African Americans and health care. *Am J Public Health.* 1997, 87(11):1773–1778.

5. Burney, L. E. Control of syphilis in a Southern rural area: a preliminary report. *Am J Public Health.* 1939, 29(9):1006–1014.

6. Shafer, J. K. Applied epidemiology in venereal disease control. *Am J Public Health.* 1954(3), 44:355–359.

7. Brown, W. J. Letter to the Editor. *Am J Public Health.* 1965, 55(6):809–810.

8. Potthoff, C. J. A selected public health bibliography with annotations. Thirty year follow-up on syphilis. *Am J Public Health.* 1965(3), 55:483–486.

9. Governing Council of the American Public Health Association. Resolutions and position papers. Biomedical experimentation in the institutional setting: suggestion for protection of "captive" populations. *Am J Public Health.* 1973, 63(6):545–560.

10. Thomas, S. B., and Quinn, S. C. The Tuskegee Syphilis Study, 1932 to 1972: implications for HIV education and AIDS risk education programs in the black community. *Am J Public Health.* 1991, 81(11):1498–1505.

11. Grunfeld, G. B. Dissimilarities between Tuskegee Study and HIV/AIDS programs emphasized. *Am J Public Health.* 1992, 82(8):1176.

12. Des Jarlais, D. C., and Stepherson, B. History, ethics, and politics in AIDS prevention research. *Am J Public Health.* 1991, 81(11):1393–1394.

13. Annas, G. J., and Grodin, M. A. Human rights and maternal-fetal HIV transmission prevention trials in Africa. *Am J Public Health.* 1998, 88:560–563.

14. Bayer, R. The debate over maternal-fetal HIV transmission prevention trials in Africa, Asia, and the Caribbean: racist exploitation or exploitation of racism? *Am J Public Health.* 1998, 88(4):567–570.

15. Akhter, M. N., and Northridge, M. E. Ethics in public health. *Am J Public Health.* 2002, 92:1056.

16. Mastroianni, A. C., and Kahn, J. P. Risk and responsibility: Ethics, *Grimes v Kennedy Krieger,* and public health research involving children. *Am J Public Health.* 2002, 92(7):1073–1076.

17. Buchanan, D. R., and Miller, F. G. Justice and fairness in the Kennedy Krieger Institute Lead Paint Study: The ethics of public health research on less expensive, less effective interventions. *Am J Public Health.* 2006, 96(5):781–787.

18. Krieger, N. Does racism harm health? Did child abuse exist before 1962? On explicit questions, critical science, and current controversies: an ecosocial perspective. *Am J Public Health.* 2003(2), 93:194–199.

19. Herrera, A. P., Snipes, S. A., King, D. W., Torres-Vigil, I., Goldberg, D. S., and Weinberg, A. D. Disparate inclusion of older adults in clinical trials: priorities and opportunities for policy and practice change. *Am J Public Health.* 2010, 100(4S):S105–S112.

20. Musa, D., Schulz, R., Harris, R., Silverman, M., and Thomas, S. B. Trust in the health care system and the use of preventive health services by Black and White adults. *Am J Public Health*. 2009, 99(7):1293–1299.

21. Quinn, S. C. Protecting human subjects: the role of Community Advisory Boards. *Am J Public Health*. 2004, 94(6):918–922.

22. McGrath, M. M., Fullilove, R. E., Kaufman, M. R., Wallace, R., and Fullilove, M. T. The limits of collaboration: A qualitative study of community ethical review of environmental health research. *Am J Public Health*. 2009, 99(8):1510–1514.

23. Watkins, B. X., Shepard, P. M., and Corbin-Mark, C. D. Completing the circle: A model for effective community review of environmental health research. *Am J Public Health*. 2009, 99(11):S567S577.

24. Satcher, D. CDC's first 50 years: Lessons learned and relearned. *Am J Public Health*. 1996, 86(12):1705–1708.

25. Bozeman, B., Slade, C., and Hirsch, P. Understanding bureaucracy in health science ethics: Toward a better Institutional Review Board. *Am J Public Health*. 2009, 99(9):1549–1556.

26. Whitman, S. Letter to the Editor. *Am J Public Health*. 1974, 64(2):171–172.

Essay 6

The Southern Male Placebo Study

The Good, the Bad, and the Ugly

Ronald L. Braithwaite, James Griffin, and Mario De La Rosa

As we approach the second decade of the 21st century, it is sometimes difficult to believe that not far behind is the haunting memory of one of the most racist examples of basic human rights violations in the history of scientific research, which spanned 40 years from 1932 to 1972, the Tuskegee Syphilis Study. According to Brandt, "In 1929, under a grant from the Julius Rosenwald Fund, the United States Public Health Service (PHS) conducted studies in the rural South to determine the prevalence of syphilis among blacks and explore the possibilities for mass treatment."[1] In 1931, the Great Depression ended the continuation of these USPHS treatment clinics that had been philanthropically funded by Julius Rosenwald, an owner and Chairman of the Board of the Sears & Roebuck Company. USPHS syphilologists, who had been centrally involved with the Rosenwald program, then decided to initiate a new study on syphilis in black males given the high rate of syphilis detected in the black population around Macon County, Alabama. Thus, in 1932, they began the USPHS's Study of Untreated Syphilis in the Negro Male, a study which was conducted over a forty-year period in spite of epidemiological, scientific findings, and best practice teachings that opposed the decision to withhold treatment from study participants. The Study resulted in tremendous harm to the participants including the exacerbation of physical illness and death. Thus the Tuskegee Syphilis Study is punctuated by good, bad and ugly outcomes.

The Tuskegee investigation was essentially a process that debilitated innocent victims because of their participation in a scientific investigation by denying treatment. Had the study occurred during an international conflict as in the case of World War II, the protocol would have been tantamount to the war crimes conducted at Auschwitz or other notorious German concentration camps. This was not Auschwitz. Instead it was a series of American atrocities conducted over a forty-year period. The investigators executed the study primarily in the rural areas of the South resulting in the maltreatment of over 400 African American men, many of whom died, given the withholding of a medical treatment of choice—penicillin—once it became widely available after World War II. As related via a personal conversation with Jean Bonhomme, M.D. in Atlanta, "while there is no denying that any withholding of treatment was inexcusable, penicillin was not used successfully in human subjects until 1942 and was not mass-produced until the mid-1940s. These trials were underway for over ten years when treatment with penicillin became possible. Treatment with some of the older, much less effective and more toxic anti-syphilis drugs would have been the only option during this [earlier] period."[2]

This paper examines some of the dilemmas associated with the nation's having experienced this scientific tragedy, and it raises some questions about whether the Tuskegee Syphilis Study, or a similar experiment, could take place again in the 21st or 22nd centuries. What would be the signs, and how can we prevent the reenactment of such racism, targeted at unsuspecting disenfranchised ethnic minorities?

A continuing question associated with the investigation was how it was possible for the researchers to justify their consciences that harming people for the sake of scientific knowledge was an acceptable practice. Perhaps that is the crux of the problem that we could face today. During the Tuskegee period, African American males from rural Alabama—poor, uneducated, marginalized, and disenfranchised—held little value in the eyes of the researchers. Their lives were cheap. Losing a few African American men for the sake of the advancement of scientific knowledge was worth the investment in the eyes of these investigators. This form of objectification of human lives was common among many individuals in the 1920s through the 1960s. It was not until whistleblowers across the nation began to evoke greater awareness of human rights violations against minorities that this targeted mayhem toward African American men was slowed.

The cessation of the Tuskegee investigation took place largely because of intrepid public health practitioners and the professional convictions of a few individuals working in the public health arena. These individuals were brave enough to stand up and tell the story that exposed the investigation for what it really was. People like Peter Buxton (a CDC scientist), and others, risked their jobs, and in some cases perhaps their lives, in order to counteract the forces of ignorance at relatively high levels in the public health research community. At the very least they risked becoming victims of ostracism to discredit their willingness to stand up for what was right. Fortunately, due to media exposure and the highly provocative nature of the investigation, they were able to avoid denigration from the most prominent public health power brokers of the time.

One critical question that the Tuskegee study raises is how was it possible for researchers who were ostensibly well-educated to take such a myopic view of the phrase "do no harm" and translate that into withholding efficacious treatments, i.e., penicillin and earlier interventions for the treatment of syphilis. A possible explanation was that these researchers were influenced by a groupthink approach, most likely the result of a mob-like mentality supported by existing social conditions at that time in order to arrive at their no-treatment decision.

> Groupthink occurs when one or two people or personality styles dominate a group's culture so completely that there is no room for those with other styles, perspectives, needs, or beliefs to get their ideas on the table. In groupthink, conformity reigns supreme. The group will make great sacrifices to simply get along and maintain the peace and harmony within. Often the group overestimates its own power and morality: what they are doing is *right*, and their track record of success is so strong that they do not consider the possibility of failure.[3]

THE GOOD

On May 16, 1997, President Clinton addressed the survivors of the infamous study that has raised questions about race and medical science for decades.[4] The president said "The United States Government did something that was wrong, deeply, profoundly, morally wrong. It was an outrage to our commitment to integrity and equality for all our citizens. We can end the silence. We can stop turning our heads away. We can look at you in the eyes and finally say on behalf of the American people what the United States Government did was shameful, and I am sorry." This apology by the president was a good thing. While this apology came 65 years late, it was a good thing.

In 1973 The National Association for the Advancement of Colored People's (NAACP's) legal representatives, led by Attorney Fred Gray, filed a class action lawsuit, and this action finally resulted in monetary relief and health care services for the victims of the Tuskegee investigation. Sen. Edward Kennedy in 1973 led the way in rewriting health education and welfare regulations that govern the conduct of federally funded research in the United States.[5] The purpose was to ensure that never again would such an egregious violation of human rights occur as a result of government-sanctioned research in the United States. In the following year, 1974, the U.S. government established the Tuskegee Health Benefit Program (THBP), and the purpose of this initiative was to redress the ill effects of the Tuskegee experiment. The last widow of the men who participated in the study, a THBP fund recipient, died in 2009.[6]

What are the implications resulting from the Tuskegee Syphilis Study for the 21st and 22nd centuries? What lessons can we learn in order to prevent this tragedy from occurring again? Can it occur again right under our noses, and without our knowledge? One of the positive outcomes of this and other examples of human rights violations in the context of human research in the United States is the implementation of institutional review boards at all major federally funded academic institutions. While these safeguard entities are an important means of human subjects protection, they are not a foolproof method for ensuring the absolute health and safety of research participants. Unfortunately, unscrupulous researchers with a callous disregard for human beings are likely to circumvent any significant human-subjects'-protection mechanisms in the interest of their personal aims. When monetary gains are at stake in the form of multimillion-dollar contracts and lucrative consultantships, it will be difficult to for some researchers to turn away from these temptations.

THE BAD

One can draw a parallel between the Tuskegee Syphilis Study and another "health care related" practice of that time, namely the practice of acquiring illegal cadavers for medical student training programs. When the practice of hands-on anatomical dissection became popular in United States medical education in the late 18th and early 19th centuries, demand for cadavers exceeded the supply. Slave bodies and thefts by grave robbers met this demand. Members of the public were aware that graves were being robbed and countered with various protective measures. Since the deterrence of grave robbing took time and money, those elements of society who were least economically and socially advantaged were the most vulnerable. Enslaved and free African Americans, immigrants, and the poor were frequently the target of grave robbing. The politically powerful tolerated this behavior except when it affected their own burial sites. Slave owners sold the bodies of their deceased chattel to medical schools for anatomic dissection. Stories of the night doctors buying and stealing bodies became part of African American folklore traditions. The physical and documentary evidence demonstrates the disproportionate use of the bodies of the poor, the black, and the marginalized in furthering the medical education of white elites. History shows that these body snatches took place in Pennsylvania, Virginia, Georgia and other states as well; all in the name of science (this was bad). There is a thin line separating the *bad* from the *ugly*.

For some segments of the African American community, their distrust of public health and health care systems which continues to this day evolved out of this intertwined, and indistinguishable, pair of medicine-related bad events. The younger generation of African Americans and other ethnic minorities may not clearly understand the damaging impact of the Tuskegee Syphilis Study. The daily struggle that many of these young men and women confront today in trying to live a good life may make them oblivious to the historical implications of these events for the ongoing contemporary threat they still pose. Such is the case despite the fact that many of them understand that perhaps some factions of American society continue to hold on to the belief that some lives are not worthy of saving.

THE UGLY

The historical pharmaceutical research done with prison inmates with little to no consent was ugly, and the racism that exists relative to ethnic minorities not being treated fairly on lists to receive organ donations is ugly. Karma is a law of moral causation. This Hindu principle maintains that every act done, no matter how insignificant, will eventually return to the doer with equal impact. Good will be returned with good, while evil will be returned with evil. All of these ugly acts have a way of coming back on the perpetrators.

Movie productions illustrating the gravity of the Tuskegee Syphilis Study like *Miss Evers' Boys*, although helpful, may not have been a sufficient source of education to reach the required number of individuals in ethnic minority communities. We need additional media venues that will educate our society about the important benefits of human subjects protection. If these efforts are not undertaken, the sacrifice of African American men, women, and children to scientific investigation may be just as much of a threat now as it was in the past. Without overemphasizing the threat, what assurances exist in our world society, which now prides itself on its ability to prevent human subject's abuses, that all will remain true to a high ethical standard in the conduct of scientific research? At the same time, new enlightenment and sensitivity to human rights violations is taking place in the midst of reports about worldwide sale of human internal organs and other body parts—an ugly act. The sale of organs and other body parts results from, and is primarily due to, scientific advancements that our global society has made in the deployment of technologies for improving the human condition. The transplantation of heart and lungs have become commonplace everywhere on the globe. However, we lack the technology for instilling "good" into the hearts of some researchers today who remain mired in thinking as if they were living in the dark ages. Human life in the minds of some researchers appears to this day to still have little or no value when pitted against the almighty research dollars, Euros, pesos, etc.

SUMMARY

Let us bring this discussion home. Think about this. When one considers the HIV/AIDS epidemic, how do we know that that in a hypothetical world, an agent that totally eliminates the virus in the body is not already locked away in a university lab somewhere on the globe? This may sound like paranoia about genocide, but the incentive for maintaining prescription drugs on the market by denying world access to a cure would be enormous. It would be more lucrative in this scenario to treat AIDS as a chronic condition with a palliative treatment. Billions of dollars annually may be at stake with the denial of the cure for AIDS being comparable to withholding penicillin for the treatment of syphilis.

Further, to what degree is the American public, not to mention underserved urban communities, subject to what one might consider a grand de facto experiment driven by economic factors? Examples include the introduction of inadequately tested compounds in the national food supply without adequate regard for the interactive effects of different chemical additives. While a food additive may be innocuous by itself, when it intermingles with a separate ingested ingredient in the human body, its effect may be harmful. The number of combinations of these additives in the body may be too large and costly to examine in a rigorous scientific investigation. There is a failure to take into account airborne interactions from environmentally spread compounds through skin contact that were never designed to interact with ingested prescriptions and chemicals in the food supply. Equally problematic is the incentive to introduce unsafe drugs or consumer products to the market while concealing the potential harm that these products can yield. What about genetically engineered foods that involve the introduction of animal genes, for example, into plant specimens? With the introduction of thousands of cosmetic products on the market annually, can the American people feel safe, and if that's the case, what about the safety of inner-city residents? Do we really understand the long-term health effects of these commodities? The question for some is to some is whether minorities are more likely to be exposed to these compounds. Some would say, "Yes, they are."

With that being said, some drug manufacturers may overlook side effects and adverse events in research subjects who are prisoners. During clinical trials or after the products reach the market manufacturers may take calculated risks if the possibility of public exposure is negligible. How would today's African American males from the rural South know whether they were the object of exploitation? Would the local community be any more of a source of protection than it was during the forty-year Tuskegee period? It would be great to think otherwise—that the rural areas of society are more humane and sensitive to their potential role in aiding unethical scientific investigations. Is this situation much different from what the Tuskegee Syphilis Study participants experienced? Given the current economic challenges that United States citizens are experiencing, the motivation to support the research for economic reasons may be great enough to cause some rural, or urban for that matter, research collaborators to compromise their ethical standards.

In the final analysis, fighting the dual forces of greed and indifference toward the value of human life may continue to be the most significant obstacles to the protection of ethnic minorities in the 21st century and in the era that follows. Perhaps one of the counteracting influences needed to prevent this exploitation is a return to community empowerment in which the goal is to indoctrinate disenfranchised populations to the health threats associated with scientific research, especially in rural areas. While university-based scientific research may have greater oversight than privately funded research, commercial research may not always have the same level and quality of oversight and scrutiny. Thus the proliferation of community-based IRBs is a positive movement to protect the interests of human subjects.

Another concern from an ethical point of view is the denial of health care itself to as many of 40 million Americans. Is this practice reasonable when a sizable proportion of the populace has little or no access to preventive or remedial care? Decision makers who follow a systems philosophy recognize the interconnectedness of various elements of American society regardless of whether one considers socioeconomic status or not. The denial of health care on a macro level is hardly any different from denying available medical treatment to over 400 African American men.

Health care needs to be made more available and affordable. One of the major shortcomings of the present health care system is that while the uninsured are lawfully required to be treated in emergency rooms, these are often the most expensive sites of service delivery. In the Tuskegee Syphilis Study, however, the participants were told falsely that they were being treated, and thereby were denied the opportunity, likelihood aside, to seek treatment elsewhere. They were held in that situation and exploited as part of a medical experiment to gather data, which is different, albeit not totally, from the admittedly tragic lack of access for today's general population. Maybe the only real protection lies in nurturing the unacceptability of extreme self-interests—also known as greed—as regards desire for health care within the minority population. Perhaps it is time for ethnic minority youth to wake up, with adult support, and to understand ways to advocate for the needs of their community. This too could involve community empowerment through interactive workshops, classes, or health promotion programs.

One of the challenges that all of us face on this issue is finding ways to educate young people about the potential for exploitation in scientific investigation. Fortunately, scientific practitioners have at their disposal home- and community center–based communication systems like Skype for video conferencing. The reach of these technologies into these communities can be longer and more intense than afforded by past technology. Given the notion that "virtual education" will probably be with us for a while, systems like this can help us to gain greater saturation into remote geographical areas and into different socio-demographic market segments. This could have helped to alleviate the Tuskegee abomination if virtual technology had been in place at the time. One limitation with this approach, however, is the observation that many ethnic minority youth in a designated community still may not have access to the Internet, libraries, or other means to access virtual learning centers. As ugly as some aspects of the subject may be, key elements of human subjects protection *must* become a mandatory part of public and private education. Again, in this case, community residents must join forces to ensure that young people of all racial and ethnic backgrounds hear the whole story and that vulnerable groups understand effective ways to protect themselves from exploitation. No one else would have the same level of investment in the success of these public education–based approaches. Whether the future outcome from the legacy of the Tuskegee study is good, bad, or ugly is ultimately the responsibility of "We the People."

Ronald L. Braithwaite, PhD, is an educational psychologist and professor in the Departments of Community Health and Preventative Medicine and Psychiatry at Morehouse School of Medicine. He has held faculty appointments at Virginia Commonwealth University, Hampton University, Howard University, Rollins School of Public Health of Emory University and the School of Public Health at the University of Cape Town, South Africa. His research involves HIV intervention studies with juveniles and adults in correctional systems, social determinants of health, health disparities and community capacity building. His research spans the globe to Africa, where he has conducted HIV prevention projects.

James P. Griffin Jr., PhD (research associate professor in the Department of Community Health and Preventive Medicine at Morehouse School of Medicine), is trained in community and organizational psychology. Much of his work has been in collaboration with community-based organizations including violence, substance abuse, HIV, and hepatitis prevention initiatives. He also has experience providing programs for inmates returning to the community. His NIH-funded substance abuse and violence prevention program was career- and resiliency-based and involved African American males. He is the founder and convener of the Metropolitan Atlanta Violence Prevention Partnership (MAVPP) and recipient of multiple community service awards.

Mario De La Rosa, PhD, is a professor at the Robert Stemple College of Public Health and Social Work, Florida International University (FIU). He received his doctorate from Ohio State University and has written more than 80 scholarly publications on Latino substance abuse and HIV and other underserved populations. His career is highlighted by his effort to bring about a reduction in health disparities in our nation by working together with other researchers across the country. Dr. De La Rosa has also received funding from NIH on numerous occasions and served on numerous national scientific review panels' advisory councils.

NOTES

1. Brandt, A. M. Racism and Research: The Case of the Tuskegee Syphilis Study. *Hastings Center Magazine,* Institute of Society, Ethics and the Life Sciences, New York, NY, 1978.

2. Personal communication, Jean Bonhomme, M.D., August 2010 .

3. Fernandez, C. P. Creating thought diversity: The antidote to Groupthink. *Journal of Public Health Management Practice,* 13(6), 670–672, 2007.

4. Gray, F. D. *The Tuskegee Syphilis Study: An Insider's Account of the Shocking Medical Experiment Conducted by Government Doctors against African American Men.* Black Belt Press, Montgomery, AL, 1998.

5. Jones, J. H. *Bad Blood: The Tuskegee Syphilis Experiment.* The Free Press: New York, NY. 1993.

6. Reverby, S. M. *The Infamous Syphilis Study and Its Legacy: Examining Tuskegee.* The University of North Carolina Press: Chapel Hill, 2009.

Essay 7

Intent

The Key that Unlocks the Search for the Legacy of the USPH Syphilis Study at Tuskegee

Luther S. Williams and Monique M. Williams

The nation's longest longitudinal observational research study, a study of untreated syphilis in African American men residing in medically, socially, and economically underserved Macon County, Alabama, is the most egregious exemplar of research misconduct in our nation's history. The study demonstrates the persistence and pervasiveness of racism, deception, and exploitation in medicine and research. African American men of Macon County were encouraged to enroll for treatment of "bad blood." Rather than being treated, they were observed through the course of disease progression to death and autopsy.

The United States government, via its Public Health Service (PHS), presumably acting on the behalf of the American people, conceived, designed, funded, conducted and sustained the study for four decades. That the actual ending of the study was occasioned by its exposure by a national press report, as contrasted with a voluntary decision initiated by the PHS, is profoundly problematic. Succinctly stated, the PHS's termination of the study was a fortuitous act; hence, arguably, the cessation of the Study was, in the language of ethics, a nonvoluntary act. The consequence of this nonvoluntary action is enormous; it leaves unaddressed—even today—an understanding of the full and comprehensive intent of the study, including the motives for, and objectives of, the study.

Documents indicate that the study was initially intended as a brief (6 months to a year) study.[1,2] The intents/motives that converted a brief study to a 40-year project remain unclear. The salient issue in question is simple; absent public outcry occasioned by national press reports, for what duration and for what purposes would the study have been extended? Until the completion of autopsies of the 74 "study participants" who were still alive in 1972? For a decade longer? For another 40-year period—i.e., a repeat of the deceptive, observational study of the progression of syphilis (late latent syphilis to postmortem) with another cadre of African American men? Even longer? Ad infinitum?

In this regard, it is remarkable that the Health Education and Welfare (HEW) Tuskegee Study Ad Hoc Advisory Panel's Final Report[3] did not address this seemingly unavoidable, self-evident issue. While, the HEW panel engaged in a substantive examination of "whether the study was justified in 1932," "should penicillin have been provided when it became available in the early 1950s," and other issues, that the panel neglected to determine and report the overall intent of the study, inclusive of its duration, borders on the incomprehensible.

Is the question of whether the study was justified in 1932 of greater saliency than its justification one year later or a decade, or two or four decades later, and can one even answer this question without gaining clarity as regards its intent? The fact that the panel even considered the issue of whether penicillin should have been provided when it became available for a study of untreated syphilis impresses one as absurd. For, by any essential definition of a study of "untreated syphilis," the issue was moot! Moreover, the report of a subsequent U. S. Senate hearing on the Study,[4] otherwise replete with inquiries by the Senate committee members directed to the "study participants" (victims), is decidedly silent on this fundamental issue of the intent of the study. Did the Committee expect the "study participants" (apparently having been asked to serve as "informed substitutes" for the PHS officials who conducted the study) who did not even know that they were involved in the research study or know the nature/intent of the study per se to answer any questions of substance or investigative utility?

There was a development that appears to offer a possible answer to this core issue of intent, including the planned endpoint of the study: namely, a Center for Disease Control (CDC) Committee voted in 1969 (37 years post initiation of the study) to continue the study absent specifying its end point.[5] Given this CDC decision, is it reasonable to assume that the planned end point of the study was three years hence (1972)? Thus, while the question remains definitively unanswered, the sheer force of logic compels one to inexorably surmise that the PHS would have extended the Study beyond 1972. Moreover, while the formal engagement of the "study participants" ended in 1972–1973, the assumption that the "study" of biological samples collected prior to death and at autopsy ceased and the samples were archived and/or destroyed by a group of professionals who appeared to have employed any and all means, including deception and coercion, to sustain the study requires a disposition at variance with rational thought. The key summary point is that the study was presumably conducted with a high level of intentionality that served to define its overall objective, investigative protocol and sampling requirements and, lastly, duration, although the duration might reasonably have been iteratively determined over the long expanse of time. However, such is not the question. The question is: what was its intended duration and why? Thus, can the legacy of the Study be rendered fully explicit absent a definitive answer to this critically important question bearing on PHS motive or intent? Even acknowledging the plethora of publications bearing on other aspects of the study,[5,6,7] in our view, the answer to this profoundly important question remains a resounding no!

To place the study in its appropriate context, we begin our search for the intent and motives of the study within two of the original scientific publications as provided by the investigators themselves.[1,2] The titles of those two articles speak to "Untreated Syphilis in the Negro Male." What exactly does this mean? Untreated syphilis means exactly that which is conveyed by the two words. The Study's title connotes the investigators' intent to pursue a longitudinal, observational study without planned therapeutic interventions. Thus, as regards the investigative design and sampling and analysis protocols, this observational study would have consisted of (a) initial diagnostic tests to confirm the existence of latent (secondary) syphilis, (b) iterative collection of samples (primarily via lumbar puncture [spinal tap] for diagnosis of neurosyphilis), and (c) assessment of later stage progression of syphilis and, importantly, summative pathological analyses of cardiovascular and neurological destruction during the postmortem examination. Since the study was (a) conducted as an observational study in design (apparently the study methods did not offer the capacity to control for the impact of larger environmental factors, inclusive of the complications to the study occasioned by the onset of other diseases); (b) employed a rather irregular and casual schedule, as described by the investigators, for "herding" the participants for testing, examinations, and sample collection (major examinations and sampling being only performed in 1939, 1948, 1963, and 1970); and (c) used a rather "elastic definition of "controls" for the study, it is hardly distinguished by its procedural specificity and intellectual rigor. In addition to the apparent and well-known ethical transgressions of the research team, the investigators developed a study fraught with design flaws and methodological missteps that meant that the study by definition could yield little of the relevant data it was intended to provide.

The study, as initiated in 1932, can be understood as an observational research project in which physician scientists served as witnesses to the progression of disease with detrimental and potentially lethal sequelae. Physicians in this era benefited from the guidance of the Hippocratic Oath and its relevant admonitions regarding appropriate care of patients. Thus, these physician scientists deviated from the basic tenets of their profession, ignoring beneficence, nonmaleficence, and justice, i.e., the study entailed observing the progression of a potentially fatal disease in a specific cohort in nature, where "nature" was the persistent dehumanizing and inhumane plantation environment of the Jim Crow–era South (as contrasted with individuals observed in a carefully defined clinical research environment) with the singular intervention being the prevention of the individuals from encountering, procuring and consuming products of known efficacy as regards the disease in question. For such a study, issues such as the administration of penicillin or other treatments that were available were—in two words—absurdly irrelevant, as it was consciously designed as an intentional study of untreated syphilis! That the above characterization is accurate is affirmed by the published findings and words of the PHS officials who conducted the study in their 14 scientific papers that were published during the duration of the study.[5] Shockingly, this series of 14 papers in reputable medical journals over the study's 40-year duration suggests that this study must have been condoned by the medical community at large, who via these publications had full opportunity to be aware of the study and its design. Unfortunately, and less than scientifically, the study investigators never did provide their protocol, which could have illuminated further the motivations and intended outcomes of the study.

In their 1936 paper, Raymond A. Vonderlehr and colleagues indicated that determining the effectiveness of treatment for syphilis and the impact of treatment on prevention of late effects of the disease have considerable public health implications.[2] The authors indicated that the "material included in this study consists of 399 syphilitic male Negroes who had never received treatment, 201 nonsyphilitic Negro males, and 275 male Negroes who had been given treatment during the first two years of the syphilitic process." It is noteworthy, in the negative, that the paper indicates that a comparison group of individuals who had received some treatment for syphilis was included in the initial analyses. In a section entitled "Morbidity in Untreated Syphilis" the authors delineate the adverse consequences of untreated syphilis. In a comparison of men with and without syphilis aged 25 to 39 years, men with syphilis had a fivefold higher rate of cardiovascular disease, and for men 40 years and older, the rate of cardiovascular disease was nearly two times higher for men with syphilis. Diseases of the central nervous system were ten times higher in men with syphilis (26.1% vs. 2.5%). When individuals with untreated syphilis were compared to those who received partial or inadequate treatment, the results are equally alarming. Therefore, for a comparison group inadequately treated for the disease, there are markedly lower rates of morbidity of advanced syphilis. The authors suggest that a 20-year period of observation would be need to fully understanding the impact of untreated syphilis. However, the baseline data presented provide compelling and sufficient evidence of the disease's impact. Any study conducted presently that demonstrated such a marked difference in outcomes would have been halted and treatment initiated.

If the primary objective of the study was to prove that treatment for syphilis was necessary, this paper, published early in the course of the study demonstrated the morbidity conferred by the untreated disease. The barbarity attending this observational study is evidenced in words attributed to PHS Study officials that further evidence the nature of the Study include: "As I see it, we have no further interest in the patients until they die"; and, "We now know, where we could only have surmised before, that we have contributed to their ailment and shortened their lives."[8]

In addition, in a sustained process akin to the activities of slave bounty hunters of a prior era, the PHS sought to "recapture" and thereby prevent the "study participants" from receiving treatment for syphilis at sites beyond the immediate control of the PHS.[8] That the PHS was apparently successful in this disgusting enterprise, one whose reach extended from Alabama to several Southeastern and Midwestern communities to which some "study participants" had relocated, serves to redefined the "place" of the horrific transactions from Macon County, Alabama, alone to other parts of the state of Alabama and even regional sites, at least as regards the maintenance of a state of untreated syphilis.

Lastly, we observe that despite the overwhelming documentation that untreated syphilis was the defining element of the study, in a most disingenuous statement uttered upon public revelation of the Study, one that occupies rare placement in the annals of human history, a PHS official observed that "subjects were informed that they could get treatment for syphilis any time; participants were not denied drugs; rather, they were not offered drugs."[4,8] The PHS official, we note, made a statement which in fact connotes "a distinction without a difference," hence, it is balderdash.

What is the significance of the last few words of the Study title, "in the Negro Male in Macon County, Alabama"? Do these words simply afford precision as regards "study participant" identification and geographic placement? We think not! As has been excellently explicated, the engagement of these men in the study was a logical derivative of long history of vile and abusive exploitation of African Americans in "medical experimentation," measured from the era of legally mandated slavery to Jim Crow–premised apartheid and beyond.[7,8] Notably, among the legal and sociopolitical machinations that served as the anchors for such heinous activities are the U.S.

Supreme Court rulings in *Dred Scott v. Sandford* and and *Plessy v. Ferguson.*[9,10] In *Dred Scott,* Justice Taney's majority opinion was infamous and the racial animus and sentiments expressed in that opinion arguably reflected the racial sentiments of the larger society in the mid-19th century and, we submit, well into the 20th century.

Specifically, as the *Dred Scott* case considered blacks to be "inferior" and "property," it is, thus, reasonable to assume that the same racial animus and sentiment were reechoed in the Syphilis Study by the researchers, at least upon its initiation. *Plessy v. Ferguson* institutionalized de jure segregation, which both approved and enabled the robust implementation of the Jim Crow segregation system in the South. The on-the-ground consequences of these two court rulings, taken in combination with the sentiments attending social Darwinism, white paternalism, the stringently enforced restriction of education and human development programs benefiting African Americans, major instances of extreme poverty, the nearly absoluteness of a plantation-based economy and, more generally, the employment of African Americans under conditions characterized by little to no compensation,[13] equal a rare opportunity of "medical experimentation" on those persons massively oppressed by the aforementioned socio-political and economic system. Add to the above vulgar mix the regularity of savage acts of violence that serve to terrorize the African American population[11] and one can imagine the foul cloud of racism that hovered over Macon County, Alabama, in the early 1930s. It, thus, became an "ideal," but definitively not a unique southern U.S. site for the PHS Study. That the Study categorically focused on African American men is consistent with their placement on the lowest rung of America's racial hierarchy, a matter that we view as unrelated to residence in Macon County, Alabama, per se.

Thus, what of the legacy of this Syphilis Study? As we understand it, legacy refers to some event/undertaking that is important to recall/has resonance for/impacts current events, undertakings and actions—collective or individual. In this regard, it is accurate to conclude that, upon the public discovery of this morally despicable study, the U.S. government halted it and there is every reason to assume that it was of constructive utility in the formulation of guidelines and standards for the conduct of research human subject research, i.e., the Belmont Report, various Department of Health and Human Service/National Institutes of Health(HHS/NIH) policy statements and requirements.[12,13] Thus, in this regard, its impact on current activities is salutary.

Another dimension of the legacy of the Study is its lingering impact on African American attitudes regarding participation in biomedical research, clinical trials in particular. For this matter, there is both a paradox and a consequence-domain limit. First, the paradox: given the growing epidemic of health disparities affecting the African American community, it is crucially important that African Americans be included in noteworthy clinical trials. And recent reports evidencing a more favorable trust-to-distrust ratio and increased African American participation in important clinical trials are encouraging. However, analysis of some the published reports bearing on this issue suggests that, in some instances, African Americans' participation in human subject research is not based on personal and full understanding of informed consent (emphasis being assigned to the participant's knowledge/ understanding as contrasted with explanations provided by the biomedical researchers). To the extent to which such is accurate and widespread, the possibility of the present/future becoming a repeat of the past, at least in part, looms as a possibility.

Regarding the consequence-domain limit, there is no plausible reason to assume that extant African American attitudes/dispositions regarding human participation in medical research are owing entirely to the Syphilis Study. To reach such a conclusion requires negation of the American history of medical experimentation on blacks, in general.[14] Thus, is the objection to participation in such research based on the Syphilis Study or the American racism that the enabled the Syphilis study? This is not a trivial question; to address the matter effectively would appear to obligate acknowledging the difference.

There remain two elements of this reflection that we view as quite problematic in the current context. While potential human participants are advantaged by the aforementioned policies and standards that are intended to uniformly govern practice, the legacy of the Syphilis Study is relevant. Do such governing conditions necessarily yield the desired action/behavior? While there were no such specific overarching regulations/declarations in 1932, it undeniable that the PHS physicians/biomedical scientists who conducted the study were also not impacted by (fully ignored) the emergence of the Nuremberg Code in the late 1940s nor the World Health Association adoption of the Declaration of Helsinki in 1964.They even ignored the societal transformative events occasioned by the civil rights movement, the Civil Rights Act of 1964, and the Voting Rights Act of 1965. In this study, the level of deception and blatant lies of the PHS investigators rendered matters such as therapeutic/nontherapeutic research, informed consent, and even "uninformed consent" imaginary. While submitting voluntarily to serve as a "study participants" did not constitute consent, we found no evidence of voluntary participation in the actual study that was being conducted, i.e., the observation of untreated syphilis. In sum, the Study stands as an abject lesson of that which can occur, even for years, declaration, policies and larger societal transformations notwithstanding.

In conclusion, the last matter (element) is that which represents the core of this essay. We simply insist that understanding the full impact of the study on contemporary activities obligates answering the question initially posited. To reiterate, we are not inquiring about some nebulous linguistic constructs or semantic variable bearing on deeply held private motives of the PHS investigators, about which one could easily engage in misrepresentation. Straightforwardly, and to reiterate, the issue is as follows: (a) the study, albeit observational, was conducted for decades; (b) it was halted nonvoluntarily by a decision of an external body; and (c) since, even this poorly executed study must have had an intent (a course of action one intended to follow, a prescribed purpose, something one planned to do/the end one sought, the goal one set to accomplish) with a defined time frame, we ask what was the overall intent of the Study and for what duration? We suggest that an important dimension of the legacy of the study is this critically important question, which to our knowledge, remains unanswered!

Luther S. Williams, PhD (distinguished professor of biology, dean of graduate studies and research, and provost and vice president for academic affairs, Tuskegee University) is a molecular biologist whose basic research has focused on the control of gene expression for the majority of his 41-year career. More recently his work has addressed underrepresentation of minorities in science and engineering and he presently directs a NIH-funded bioethics infrastructure initiative focused bioethics training. He has served as a member of the National Center (Institute) for Minority Health Disparities Advisory Council and currently serves as a member of the NIH Director's Council.

Monique M. Williams, MD, MSCI (assistant professor of medicine and psychiatry, Division of Geriatrics and Nutritional Science, Washington University School of Medicine), serves as the director of the Community Outreach and Recruitment Core of the NIH-funded Bioethics Infrastructure Initiative. Her principal research focuses on Alzheimer's disease in African Americans and minority participation in clinical trials.

NOTES

1. R. A. Vonderlehr, T. Clark, and J. R. Heller. 1936. Untreated Syphilis in the Male Negro: A Comparative Study of Treated and Untreated Cases. *JAMA*. 107:856–860.

2. R. A. Vonderlehr et al. 1936. "Untreated Syphilis in the Male Negro: A Comparative Study of Treated and Untreated Cases. *Venereal Disease Information*. 17:260–265.

3. Tuskegee Syphilis Study Ad Hoc Panel to Department of Health, Education and Welfare, 1973. Final Report. Superintendent of Documents, Washington, D.C.

4. S. M. Reverby (ed.). "Tuskegee's Truths: Rethinking the Tuskegee Syphilis Study." *Testimony of Four Survivors from the United States Senate Hearings on Human Experimentation*. University of North Carolina Press, Chapel Hill, 2000.

5. S. Bell. "Events in Tuskegee Syphilis Study" pp. 34–38, in S. M. Reverby (ed.), *Tuskegee's Truths: Rethinking the Tuskegee Syphilis Study.* University of North Carolina Press, Chapel Hill, 2000.

6. T. L. Beauchamp and L. Walters. *Contemporary Issues in Bioethics.* 394–401, Wadsworth. 2003.

7. V. N. Gamble. 1997. "Under the Shadow of Tuskegee: African Americans and Health Care." *Amer. J. of Public Health,* 87:1773–1778.

8. S. M. Reverby. *Examining Tuskegee: The Infamous Syphilis Study and its Legacy.* University of North Carolina Press, Chapel Hill, 2009.

9. A. L. Allen and T. Pope. "Social Contract Theory, Slavery and Antebellum Courts" in *A Companion to African American Philosophy.* T. L. Potts and J. L. Pittman (eds.). Blackwell Publishing, 2006.

10. H. McGary. "The Legacy of *Plessy v Ferguson.*" In *A Companion to African American Philosophy.* T. L. Potts and J. L. Pittman (eds.). Blackwell Publishing, 2006.

11. D. A. Blackmon. *Slavery by Another Name: The Re-Enslavement of Black People in America from the Civil War to World War II.* Doubleday, 2008.

12. National Commission for the Protection of Human Subjects of Biomedical and Behavioral Research (National Commission) 1979. Belmont Report: Ethical Principles and Guidelines for the Protection of Human Subjects of Research. Washington, D.C.; U.S. Government Printing Office.

13. NIH Guidelines on the Inclusion of Women and Minorities as Subjects in Clinical Research. National Institutes of Health. NIH Guide. 1994 23:2–3.

14. H. A. Washington. *Medical Apartheid: The Dark History of Medical Experimentation on African Americans from Colonial Times to the Present.* Doubleday, Random House, Inc. New York. 2006.

Essay 8

The Untold Story of the Legacy of the Tuskegee Study of Untreated Syphilis in the Negro Male

Or, Is the Legacy of Tuskegee Affirmative Action for White Researchers?

Vickie M. Mays

The prevailing legacy of the Tuskegee Study of Untreated Syphilis in the Negro Male has evolved to be the mistrust by African Americans of participation in scientific research studies.[1-2] This view of the skepticism of African Americans to participate in the research enterprise based on mistrust developed as a function of the Tuskegee Study of Untreated Syphilis in The Negro Male has been widely studied, written about and held as the cause or blame for the lack of success in addressing particular health disparities in African Americans. This view is held despite the growing number of studies documenting that a number of African Americans have little to no knowledge of the events of Tuskegee, that their willingness to participate in research is not directly or indirectly connected to the events of the study and expressed willingness to be members of research studies depending on the conditions and nature of the research.[3-11] Medical historians have pointed out on various occasions that the mistrust of science and health pre-dates the Tuskegee Study of Untreated Syphilis in The Negro Male.[12-14] This myth of unwillingness to participate in research by African Americans continues in the face of two challenging facts about African American participation in research. The first is the growth in the actual numbers of African American participants in the research enterprise (post the NIH mandatory requirement of inclusion of racial/ethnic minorities). The second is also the increase in the numbers of large African American cohort studies under the supervision of both minority and non-minority Principal Investigators (e.g. Jackson Heart Study, ARIC, AASK).[15-18]

This raises the question, in the face of growing numbers of studies which document that mistrust in research is *not* the overwhelming factor affecting African American participation in the research enterprise, [12–14] of who benefits from the perpetuation of mistrust as the legacy of the Tuskegee Study of Syphilis in The Untreated Negro Male? Reverby has discussed a number of alternative ways of thinking about the metaphor of the Tuskegee Study of Untreated Syphilis in The Negro Male[12–14,19] but the legacy of mistrust is enduring.

Myths and misappropriations exist for reasons and often support beliefs and agendas. There are several potential beneficiaries as well as those who are potentially harmed by the legacy of mistrust. The most significant harm is using the difficulty of engaging African Americans in the research enterprise as an explanation for the lack of progress in health equity in the United States. It is the United States where a black man in Harlem at the end of the 20th century was more likely to die young than a person in Bangladesh.[20] Former Surgeon General Satcher examined mortality rates and found that between 1991 and 2000, African Americans compared to whites lost more than 800,000 lives because of inequities.[21] Those who are accountable for the development of the science necessary to resolve these disparities benefit from the perspective that African Americans' lack of cooperation in research is partially responsible for their health disparities.

In examining the NIH Reporter for grants with the explicit goal to study the Tuskegee Study of Untreated Syphilis in The Negro Male's impact on mistrust in African Americans, the majority of the principal investigators of these NIH grants were nonminority. The exceptions were one African American and a second whose racial identity could not be verified by Internet searches. Beneficiaries are also the authors of publications that promote the legacy of mistrust by African Americans in the research enterprise. Examining several of these publications especially in the area of implications for HIV research, these authors conclude that the lack of participation by African Americans in their studies is a function of mistrust based on the legacy of Tuskegee. Striking is how few of these articles gave serious examination to their methods and procedures or proposed other more compelling contributing factors for the difficulty that they encountered in getting African Americans to participate in HIV research. HIV is one of the research topics that functions in the shadow of a history of forced sterilizations, perceived genocide, racialized, controlled and contested sexuality ranging from black male masculinity to the ownership of the bodies of black women during slavery. Yet despite the divisive historical memories that are raised in HIV research, little are these historical events evoked in comparison to the use of Tuskegee as the basis for failure to enroll African Americans in HIV research.[22] While in most instances it is nonminorities who benefit from the mistrust legacy there are a few racial/ethnic minorities who also keep alive mistrust as the legacy of the Tuskegee Study. NIH/CDC funding to develop educational efforts on how to conduct research in a manner that overcomes this legacy of mistrust, along with anticipated publications are real and tangible benefits for those who keep astir the myth of mistrust.

TEACHING AND TRAINING TO DO RESEARCH VS DOING RESEARCH

In 1993, the National Institutes of Health (NIH) passed The Revitalization Act which mandated that all NIH funded clinical trials have "appropriate representation" of minority and women participants.[23] Four years later in the 1997 Tuskegee Apology[25] President Clinton called for the training of researchers in bioethics so that what happened with men who participated in the Tuskegee Study of Untreated Syphilis in the Negro Male would not happen again.

While the NIH mandate for the inclusion of racial and ethnic minorities was a step in the right direction, also needed was a population based racial/ethnic/culturally informed bioethics and research methodology training in academic institutions that would ensure that researchers would have the necessary foundations to conduct ethical research within racial/ethnic minority populations. NIH, post the 1997 Tuskegee Apology, has invested heavily in extramural/intramural research ethics trainings designed to meet President Clinton's call to action.[26–27] Following Clinton's Apology, between 1999–2009 NIH funded 29 short-term research ethics courses through the T15 program. My T15 "Research Ethics in Biomedical and Behavioral Research in Racial/Ethnic Minority Populations" ethics course was designed for academic researchers and CEOs of community organizations whose agencies were regularly accessed as research sites by universities and medical centers. Ten independent modules were designed that examine (through case studies, lectures, interactive activities and community-partner-led sessions) how the research enterprise—ranging from research designs, statistical approaches, communication of findings to the maintenance of biological samples—could put specific racial/ethnic subpopulations at risk for harm.

The completion of a culturally driven informed consent was a requirement along with a twenty-page manuscript on some aspect of harm, beneficence or identification of an unique IRB community concern. The course was designed not only to help researchers understand harm as it potentially affects the individual but also to understand the intricate way the individual's common fate and less than six degrees of separation are often tied to community and family as a function of vulnerabilities based on gender, race, class, place, age and historical relationships with societal institutions.[23] While mine and a few of the other T15s go beyond the mere retelling of the story of the Tuskegee Study of Untreated Syphilis in The Negro Male and focus on population based public health ethics specific to racial/ethnic minority populations, the real problem is that for many of these T15's they are not a required part of doctoral or master's level education.[27] *NIH is encouraged as part of its requirement for those who participate in its funded research that a consensus meeting be held to determine the body of knowledge necessary to reduce harm and master population based culturally informed public health research ethics. NIH should specify within its required research training specific racial/ethnic and culturally domains that must be mastered in order to be in compliance with its training in bioethics research.* Requiring competency in population-based research ethics focused on racial/ethnic minority populations would constitute a meaningful step toward the prevention of a repeat of the Tuskegee Study of Untreated Syphilis in The Negro Male.

Mastery of research ethics competency and the urgency by which it is embraced underlies the basic issue of what, in today's society, is the value of the lives of African Americans in the United States? How urgent is it that African Americans be full participants in our research enterprise? Are we really committed to participation in research for African Americans so that they may gain benefit as a group in order to address and enhance their health status and health outcomes? If the answers are uniformly yes, then we cannot tolerate "do overs" in research, where we don't have sufficient number of African Americans participating in our studies for powered analyses of their data, as time is lost in the transmission of disease and saving of lives.

We are 30 years into the HIV epidemic which disproportionately affects African Americans.[24] For every HIV research study that fails to reach African Americans or must " do over" its efforts to enroll African Americans we lose the lives of African American men and women. Even when the natural history studies recognized their lack of sufficiently powered racial/ethnic minority participation the decision was to award supplemental monies to the same group of PIs for whom data collection in these populations were low. In HIV the most defining studies for the investigative history of HIV were allowed to go on with no racial/ethnic minorities in the PI role. Even now there is not one major vaccine preparedness study that has ever been headed up by an African American as Principal Investigator despite the critically needed expertise on African Americans in order to successfully recruit, enroll and maintain them in these studies. This is not due to a lack of competent nonmajority PIs. Rather, it reflects a highly competitive NIH review system that simultaneously: 1) rewards for past history of funding (hence favoring majority investigators); 2) is marked by implicit bias of what is good science; 3) is impacted by a lack of seasoned reviewers with specialized expertise in racial/ethnic minority topics; and, 4) under-rewards for cultural competency (a factor which might reduce the need for "do overs").

There are ways in which the injustices of Tuskegee continue. I am often struck by the efforts of NIH to recruit new racial/ethnic minority investigators into the HIV/AIDS field. But NIH has yet to ask itself what happened to the early investigators it trained who toiled in the field being used as data collectors under the guise of minority supplements. All too often these investigators whose efforts in the community imbued them with valuable knowledge on cultural competency have walked away and joined other fields of research because the most major and valued studies in HIV remained in the hands of a small group of nonminority investigators. It is unfortunate that these much-needed minority investigators are not being recruited back into HIV/AIDS research.

It is the African American community who today is not doing well in their health that loses when all are tainted by the brush of "'we' don't participate in research studies." This continuation of the myth of the lack of participation at the level of NIH and CDC is of greater benefit for white researchers who are allowed budgets and time in their grant effort to learn how to conduct research in minority communities while minority investigators fail to even make the peer review grade for recommended funding. I remember the experience of sitting on a NIH standing review committee for HIV/AIDS proposals and being the only racial/ethnic minority on the committee, having to argue that a proposed recruitment strategy in a study would be ineffective and this was an indicator of the lack of knowledge of the population that would be needed for the study to be successful in reducing HIV in African Americans. I was outvoted and the study was funded. Out of interest and curiosity I watched the study from afar. The researchers with a predominantly white team and "indigenous interviewers" failed to bring in a large enough sample of African American Males who have Sex with Males (MSM) to be able to analyze the data. Yet the study team was rewarded with supplemental funding to try again. It is "do overs" of this type that add to years of life lost, mortality and morbidity. In each study we publish in which we allude to the difficulties of the population in participation in research we blame them, and not ourselves.

In my T15 course, the module on communication of research findings is taught by the community partners. Real examples are presented by the community of the negative consequences of how the media frames our research results. One such story told was of a teacher in an elementary school classroom who had a very punitive approach to gathering permission slips for the African American students because she was aware that African Americans did not participate the way others did. This punitive approach to those students was intended to get the child to gain the attention of his or her parents as the child wanted to avoid the penalties. This of course was all done for the good of the child to make sure that they would get their parents' attention to complete the permission slip. The end justified the means, as one parent was told, since it was for the good of her child.

BENIGN NEGLECT VS HISTORICAL MISTRUST

In thinking about how to prevent another Tuskegee Study of Untreated Syphilis in The Negro Male from occurring it may be less about understanding the particulars of the incident of the past than about understanding how existing vulnerabilities of racial/ethnic minority communities in today's society can result in unintended harm. Sometimes this is as simple as understanding the consequences of cash payments to a participant who is on any type of assistance program. If payment is not reported (which would then be deducted) they could be disqualified by the assistance program. Yet university accounting procedures of signing receipts and wanting Social Security numbers just increases the likelihood of a problem occurring.

It has been said that the incident of the Tuskegee Study of Untreated Syphilis in the Negro Male has gone from science to conspiracy to metaphor.[1,12-14] What's interesting is this metaphor is kept alive much more by researchers and those in professional capacities than the average African American in the community who on our surveys does not know about the Tuskegee Study of Untreated Syphilis in The Negro Male. If not Tuskegee, then what accounts for the reluctance? It is the benign neglect that occurs every day in the lives of some African Americans. It is the message that the lives of African Americans are not valued in a manner similar to those of other Americans. It is the social exclusion of African Americans' participation in society in the forms of lack of quality education, segregated housing in neighborhoods that suffer from all of the effects of poverty, lack of resources and poor public services. It is a message that is experienced by the large mass of African Americans convicted of felonies who are disenfranchised from voting. Imagine while everyone talked about their excitement about voting for the first black president that many African Americans, particularly men, could not vote. So when researchers extol the benefit of research it is yet another unmet promise that accounts for the lack of interest. Mistrust comes from years of being in studies but never getting the benefit much the way the men of the Tuskegee Study of Untreated Syphilis in The Negro Male provided data for the benefit of the health of others. These everyday experiences of neglect, benign or otherwise, are what drive the mistrust. Also, just the conditions of African Americans in this country make them more vulnerable in the research enterprise as their fate is so deeply connected to their community and each other, which is often not understood or taught when bioethics is taught at the level of the individual and not the population.

FORGOTTEN BUT POSITIVE LEGACIES OF TUSKEGEE

The real legacy of the Tuskegee Study of Untreated Syphilis in the Negro Male is yet to be told because of unfulfilled promises from President Clinton's Apology directives.[25] The directives of the Apology are opportunities missed to change not only the relationships between researchers and the racial/ethnic minority community but potentially the moral compass for research. President's Clinton's Apology was a public acknowledgment of a lack of regard, a fault, a deficit in the federal government's protection of a group of its citizens. Clinton's Apology was a means to an end and we should not by attrition of resources and changes in administration let it slowly become an end. The Apology should be viewed as the opportunity for improvement in the research community's relationships with African Americans.[7] As with any apology it can make the relationship even better than before as one human element about a sincere apology is it says, above all else, that you care about the relationship. However if the responsibility for the directives of the Apology remain in the hands of U.S. Department of Health and Human Services (DHHS) with little accountability to the White House or some entity that will be the spokesperson for black America, then conflict of interest by the DHHS for research approaches will continue to dominate. *The White House should revisit and evaluate whether the end that it hoped the Apology would reach has occurred and if not next steps to achieve the goals.*

Often overlooked are the contributions of the African American professionals in the Tuskegee study.[12–14] There are lessons of recruitment and retention that were developed within the Tuskegee Study that have gone practically unexplored and unrecognized that are cultural lessons. Describing the use of the incentive of burial insurance or other techniques that were developed could give a rightful recognition in the research enterprise of the critical importance of African American professional staff and African American cultural sensibilities in African American studies.

Why do we not celebrate the contributions of the men who participated in the Tuskegee Study of Untreated Syphilis in the Negro Male? Why do we not know their stories? What were the values, beliefs, and motivations of the men who participated in the study? We should celebrate their volunteerism much the way that we celebrate those who volunteer for war. They gave their lives not to save the country but to save other humans who were exposed to a then deadly disease. We have had many awards ceremonies and plaques for those volunteering in the fight against cancer, HIV/AIDS and any number of other diseases, but we have made the legacy of these men not about what they did but about what we have failed to do. To honor these men makes visible our shame at our behavior.

So often the study is referred to as the Tuskegee Study of Untreated Syphilis, having dropped the most important part, which is the reference to "Untreated Negro Male." This helps to hide the inhumanity of the study. It is clearly time for a new legacy, not that of mistrust but of the contributions of the men and their wives and children who are the unsung heroes who gave their lives for science.

It is also time for us to fulfill the promises of President Clinton to train researchers so that what happened in Tuskegee will never happen again. It should never happen again whether it be in an actual study that fails to provide treatment to the participants when a cure is found or research activities that are a metaphor of the disvaluing of the lives of African Americans. Currently both conditions continue as participants in HIV studies in international setting help bring a drug to market but are never able to afford the drug and die prematurely. We must ask ourselves the difficult question of what is the value of the life of an African American and do the right thing. Let us honor what happened in the Tuskegee Study of Untreated Syphilis in the Negro Male by developing a legacy of research ethics training that is population-based and public health in nature that mandates an education informed by culture, race and ethnicity for every researcher who works with African American populations as a start to truly reduce and eliminate health disparities.

Vickie M. Mays, PhD, MSPH (professor of psychology and health services, UCLA), is a clinical psychologist trained in health services and epidemiology who has published papers on research ethics in racial/ethnic minority populations. Funded by a NIH T32 she created a course on research ethics in behavioral and biomedical research in racial/ethnic minorities. Her interests in research ethics includes HIV/AIDS, ethics of research methodologies, data policies and data analytic strategies in working with African Americans and small sample populations such as American Indians. She is director of the UCLA Center on Research, Education, Training and Strategic Communication on Minority Health Disparities (www.minorityhealthdisparities.org).

NOTES

1. Thomas, S., & Quinn, S. (1991). Public Health Then and Now, The Tuskegee Syphilis Study, 1932 to 1972: Implications for HIV education and AIDS risk education programs in the black community. *American Journal of Public Health* 81, 1498–1505.

2. Shavers, V., Lynch, C., & Burmeister, L. (2000). Knowledge of the Tuskegee Study and its impact on willingness to participate in medical research studies. *Journal of the National Medical Association* 92, 563–72.

3. Katz, R., Kegeles, S., Green, B., Kressin, N., James, S., & Claudio, C. (2003). The Tuskegee Legacy Project: History, preliminary scientific findings, and unanticipated societal benefits. *Dental Clinics of North America* 47, 1–19.

4. Katz, R., Kegeles, S., Kressin, N., Green, B., Wang, M., James, S., et al. (2006). The Tuskegee Legacy Project: Willingness of Minorities to Participate in Biomedical Research. *Journal of Health Care for the Poor and Underserved* 17, 698–715.

5. Katz, R., Green, B., Kressin, N., Claudio, C., Wang, M., & Russell, S. (2007). Willingness of Minorities to Participate in Biomedical Studies: confirmatory findings from a follow-up study using the Tuskegee Legacy Project Questionnaire. *Journal of the National Medical Association* 99, 1050–1062.

6. Katz, R., Green, B., Kressin, N., Kegeles, S., Wang, M., James, S., et al. (2008). The Legacy of the Tuskegee Syphilis Study: Its Impact on Willingness to Participate in Biomedical Research Studies. *J Health Care for the Poor and Underserved* 2008; 19:1169–1181.

7. Corbie-Smith, G., Thomas, S., Williams, M., & Moody-Ayers, S. (1999). Attitudes and beliefs of African Americans toward participation in medical research. *Journal of General Internal Medicine* 14, 537–546.

8. Freimuth, V., Quinn, S., Thomas, S., Cole, G., Zook, E., & Duncan, T. (2001). African Americans' views on research and the Tuskegee Syphilis Study. *Social Science & Medicine* 52, 797–808.

9. Brown, D., & Topcu, M. (2003). Willingness to participate in clinical treatment research among older African Americans and Whites. *Gerontologist* 43, 62–72.

10. Bates, B., & Harris, T. (2004). The Tuskegee Study of Untreated Syphilis and Public Perceptions of Biomedical Research: A Focus Group Study. *Journal of the National Medical Association* 96 (8), 1051–1064.

11. Brandon, D., Issac, L., & LaVeist, T. (2005). The legacy of Tuskegee and trust in medical care: Is Tuskegee responsible for race differences in mistrust of medical care? *Journal of the National Medical Association* 97, 951–956.

12. Reverby, S. (2000). Introduction: More Than a Metaphor. Tuskegee's Truths: Rethinking the Tuskegee Syphilis Study. Chapel Hill: University of North Carolina Press 9, 8.

13. Reverby, S. (2001). More than fact and fiction. Cultural memory and the Tuskegee Syphilis Study. *Hastings Center Report* 31 (5), 22–28.

14. Reverby, S. (2009). *Examining Tuskegee: The Infamous Syphilis Study and Its Legacy.* Chapel Hill: University of North Carolina Press.

15. Wyatt, S., Diekelmann, N., Henderson, F., Andrew, M., Billingsley, G., Felder, S., et al. (2003). A community-driven model of research participation: The Jackson Heart Study Participant Recruitment and Retention Study. *Ethnicity and Disease* 13 (4), 438–455.

16. Fuqua, S., Wyatt, S., Andrew, M., Sarpong, D., Henderson, F., Cunningham, M., et al. (2005). Recruiting African-American research participation in the Jackson Heart Study: Methods, response rates, and sample description. *Ethnicity and Disease* 15 (4 Suppl 6), S6, 18–29.

17. White, A., Folsom, A., Chambless, L. E., Sharret, A., Yang, K., et al. (1996). Community surveillance of coronary heart disease in the Atherosclerosis Risk in Communities (ARIC) Study: Methods and initial two years' experience. *Journal of Clinical Epidemiology* 49 (2), 223–233.

18. Whelton, P. K., Lee, J. Y., Kusek, J. W., Charleston, J. R., DeBruge, J. B., Douglas, M. M., et al. (1996). Recruitment experience in the African American Study of Kidney disease and hypertension (AASK) pilot study. *Controlled Clinical Trials* 17, S17–S33.

19. Caplan, A. (1992). When Evil Intrudes (Twenty Years After: The Legacy of the Tuskegee Syphilis Study). *Hastings Center Reports* 22, 29–32.

20. McCord, C., & Freeman, H. (1990). Excess mortality in Harlem. *The New England Journal of Medicine* 322, 173–177.

21. Satcher, D., Fryer, G. J., McCann, J., Troutman, A., Woolf, S., & Rust, G. (2005). What if we were equal? A comparison of the black-white mortality gap in 1960 and 2000. *Health Affairs* 24 (2), 459–464.

22. Sengupta, S., Strauss, R., DeVellis, R., Quinn, S., & Ware, W. (2000). Factors affecting African-American participation in AIDS research. *Journal of Acquired Immune Deficiency Syndromes* 24, 275–284.

23. Mays, V. M. (2001). Methods for increasing recruitment and retention of ethnic minorities in health research through addressing ethical concerns. *Proceedings of the Seventh Conference on Health Survey Research Methodology* (pp. 97–99). Washington, DC: U.S.: Department of Health and Human Services, National Center for Health Statistics.

24. Mays, V. M. Ricks, J., Maas, R. M. Cochran, S. D. (2011). Changing the Future Course of the HIV Epidemic in African American Women in the U.S. South: Employing a Social Determinants Approach in Population-Level HIV Prevention and Intervention Efforts. Oxford Handbook of Health Psychology.

25. Centers for Disease Control and Prevention, Department of Health and Human Services. U.S. Public Health Service Syphilis Study at Tuskegee. Presidential Apology 1997. Available at: ⟨http://www.cdc.gov/tuskegee/clintonp.htm⟩. Accessed May 12, 2010.

26. http://bioethics.od.nih.gov/.

27. Centers for Disease Control and Prevention (1997). *U.S. Public Health Service Syphilis Study at Tuskegee. Presidential Apology 1997.* Retrieved May 12, 2010, from http://www.cdc.gov/tuskegee/clintonp.htm.

Essay 9

Legacy of Tuskegee

*Malika Roman Isler, Adebowale Odulana,
and Giselle Corbie-Smith*

TUSKEGEE AS A SYMBOL

In discussions of the Tuskegee Syphilis Study, we are often referring to a cohort of specifics: an individual study, in a designated location, with particular practices, during a set time period, with a restricted set of people. While the study was pragmatically such, the legacy of the Tuskegee Syphilis Study envelops a longer history of medical "mispractice" that precedes the period of 1932–1972 and extends well beyond this study as one of the more infamous examples of medical abuse and mistreatment in the context of research. Though for most people other examples remain nameless and their specific accounts unarticulated, many African Americans are culturally aware of the range of abuses committed against people of color in the United States during and since slavery. The Tuskegee Syphilis Study has just become the name that embodies them all.

The Tuskegee Syphilis Study has come to represent and evoke a response to a broader spectrum of social, cultural, and historical abuses experienced by racial and ethnic minorities. The name functions much like an allegory for the broader economic, health, societal, and educational inequities that many people of color experience in the United States. The epidemiological and demographic data demonstrate that, over time, more African Americans continue to live at and below the poverty level as compared to non-Hispanic whites, more are uninsured in comparison to whites, and they are disparately burdened with higher morbidity and mortality from the leading causes of illness and death. Likewise, African Americans are more likely to be incarcerated and less likely to have earned at least a high school diploma. While the Tuskegee Syphilis Study was a gross abuse that has become part of the filter for minority participation in clinical research, we offer that it alone does not shape minority involvement or even function as the predominant figure in the decision to participate. However, the Tuskegee Syphilis Study has become an epithet for the far-reaching cultural mistrust, and perhaps subconscious desire to cognitively reconcile the state of black America, that takes center stage when minorities consider participation in a largely white clinical research enterprise

PAINTING AN ACCURATE PICTURE

As part of the National Institute of Health's policy on the inclusion of women and minorities as clinical research subjects, NIH mandated that researchers address inclusion of these groups and their subpopulations in developing research designs, as appropriate to the study's objectives.[1] Guiding principles for maximizing inclusion include 1) assessing theoretical and/or scientific linkages between gender, race/ethnicity, and the study topic, 2) developing culturally appropriate outreach activities and recruitment plans, and 3) building mutually beneficial relationships between investigators and populations of interest. Even with this policy and subsequent guidelines in place, minority inclusion in clinical research has continued to lag.[2]

Participation in clinical research is influenced by awareness, access, and opportunity, all of which ultimately influence willingness to participate.[3] Despite empirical evidence indicating that minorities experience less awareness and access to clinical research opportunities, multilevel barriers, and limited facilitators, as a group they are no less willing to participate in clinical research than other ethnic or racial groups.[4-6] This remains true even in the face of well-documented historical mistrust of the clinical research institution. Katz et al. demonstrated that African Americans were more likely than whites to self-report willingness to participate in cancer screenings regardless of who performed the screening and what one was asked to do in the screening.[7] Wendler et al., in a systematic review of research enrollment decisions of approximately 70,000 individuals, found that minorities were as willing as non-Hispanic whites to participate in health research.[8]

Researcher awareness and understanding of minority willingness to participate is a significant conceptual hurdle to surmount for researchers and research institutions, but a necessary one to assume responsibility for constructing effective recruitment plans and investing in innovative and resource-intensive strategies for partnering with minority communities. Part of embracing that realization is the need to question and alter, if not outright reject, the individual and institutional-level practices and policies that allow "research as usual" from a traditional research perspective.

UNPACKING TUSKEGEE

Though the Tuskegee Syphilis Study has unquestionably become one of the most well-known abuses conducted in the name of medical research in the United States, there are several lessons to be learned that can begin to more positively shape the legacy it leaves. Despite the ethical violation of not appropriately treating participants with the best standard of care, researchers followed two approaches that all researchers in the wake of Tuskegee should consider in their work—becoming participant-centered and community-engaged. Research that is participant-centered has been hailed as an approach that fosters participation and commitment to the research process. This is largely due to the approach's focus on the needs and interests of the participant rather than the researcher,[9] which is a deviation from the way research has traditionally been done. A participant-centered approach can influence a variety of study aspects ranging from recruitment strategies to participant assignment to the dissemination strategies employed.

Even within the Tuskegee Syphilis Study, the United States Public Health Service recognized the value of meeting the salient needs of participants and capitalizing on services and outcomes that were of importance to the targeted population. While the study's outcome of interest was the natural progression of untreated syphilis, researchers provided services or incentives of interest to participants—access to free health care, free meals, and even free burial insurance.[10]

The practice of thinking beyond the professional needs of researchers and the institutional standards for conducting research allows investigators to meet recruitment goals and reframes research to become more beneficial to communities. What purpose does this research serve to the broader community? What matters to our participants? What services do they need? What changes would they like to see at the end of this study? How are they compensated for the investments they make in the research process? Each of these queries assists researchers, and even funders, in framing research agendas and the research process so that the focus is on the central figure in the study—the participant. We must also consider that, in contemporary research, a participant-centered approach should evolve out of an obligation to the moral and ethical pursuit of scientific knowledge, not as a form of coercion for covert or even overt research objectives.

The Tuskegee Syphilis Study also incorporated strategies that were community engaged. First, the study took place within the local community, alleviating the need for participants to enter the ivory tower of a medical research institution, which has largely been the approach in clinical research. Congruent with what the Tuskegee researchers recognized to be true, more communities and engaged researchers alike advocate for relocating research to where it can most easily be shaped and molded by those that it should impact the most—the communities. This has been clearly recognized for population-based studies, as is common in the socio-behavioral sciences, but is becoming more the expected norm in bench and clinical sciences with the growing popularization of consultative bodies such as community advisory boards and even clinical trials that take place outside of the large tertiary care centers. A critical evaluation of the influence of "place" for research development and engagement is a legacy lesson from Tuskegee. Considering "place" in study design is not only an opportunity to overcome the logistical and geographical barriers that can prohibit research participation, but can also be responsive to the cultural influences necessary to engage a community largely disengaged from the research process.

Among racial and ethnic minorities, community gatekeepers and opinion leaders are critical to community buy-in, endorsement, and, ultimately, engagement with research.[11] Nurse Eunice Rivers, the black nurse and study coordinator, was a face and voice with whom study participants could identify. Appropriate cultural brokers, who resonate with the identity, language, and values of a community, are essential to establishing trust and participation. Without these brokers or partners on the ground, community-engaged research will not move forward. Additionally, Nurse Rivers was brought in at beginning of the study and remained for the study's forty-year duration.

A legacy lesson to both researchers and funding institutions: engaged research requires time. Time, both in the sense of historical involvement and duration. Even with a cultural insider, time is necessary to develop the mutual trust, shared processes and products, and community participation characteristic of engaged research. The engaged process requires time investment to build and sustain the work, as well as continuity of the faces behind the work. This ongoing presence is a major foundation upon which community participation is built and is actually necessary outside the context of a study or when research is the primary focus. True engagement begins when a study is not taking place. How can researchers be of service to communities? When are we present in communities when we are not recruiting for or conducting research? What have we offered or supported within the community specific to their priorities? The time invested by partners and participants will largely mirror the time invested by the investigators and study staff.

OTHER NECESSARY CULTURAL TRANSITIONS IN RESEARCH

Regardless of how we interpret the legacy of the Tuskegee Syphilis Study, it is clear that the clinical research enterprise is making a gradual shift toward more transparency and equity in research conducted with communities. Broadly, this is through the lens of community engagement, or using a "process of working collaboratively with and through groups of people affiliated by geographic proximity, special interest, or similar situations to address issues affecting the well-being of those people."[12]

In essence, the development and conduct of research is moving beyond the confines of the research institution, both physically and conceptually. Communities are increasingly becoming not only the sites for research but also the partners, and even originators, of the intellectual research property, as well as co-owners in the governing power structures. This is appropriate in research with all communities, but particularly necessary to build bridges with communities that have a history of medical and cultural abuse and that have largely been on the languishing end of power imbalances.

By conducting research in the presence of—and in partnership with—communities, we yield the best return on investment for both communities and researchers. Full participation by both entities facilitates research that is meaningful and responsive to local community priorities, which increases buy-in and participation in the research process. Community engagement can also produce processes and products that incorporate the interpretive value of culture, and therefore have greater uptake and change in the outcomes of interest. Engaging with communities to understand and respond to issues that affect their well-being is critical to unpack the interplay of the multiple influences that create context for living. An engaged approach to research also creates the opportunity for co-learning that capitalizes on the experiences, expertise, and resources that both the research and community perspectives offer. Community engagement can vary operationally from more heavily researcher-directed models that mirror a traditional research approach to cooperative models with complete co-sharing, such as that of community-based participatory research.

The orientation and guiding principles of community engagement are a necessary cultural transition for investigators and communities to create meaningful, effective, and ethical research. However, there is also a need for a shift in the face of the clinical research enterprise, particularly as we consider the engagement of racial and ethnic minorities in the research process. While NIH has emphasized the need to support training and development of minority investigators, the number of racial/ethnic minority investigators still remains remarkably low.[1,2] An increased presence of minority investigators will benefit the research enterprise and minority communities, as minority investigators are more likely to focus on issues that disparately impact minority communities than white investigators; they often have experiences and perspectives that illuminate understanding of the critical issues underlying health disparities.[13] These diverse contributions both advance the agendas of research institutions and create more opportunities for research participation and collaboration with underrepresented partners in research—which is both our ethical and mandated charge.

A final point to consider in the wake of the Tuskegee Syphilis Study is the inherent biases in research. We attempt to achieve "truth" through a set of methodological choices and interpretive principles, however; no research is value free or neutral. All research, as the Tuskegee Syphilis Study vividly demonstrates, is reflective of the social and political norms of the time. The questions we pose, the methodologies we choose, even how we interpret our outcomes or findings are all steeped in our professional norms learned in scientific culture that reflects the thinking of the greater society. As researchers, we must practice reflexivity on our filters to become aware of how they influence the questions we pose, the populations with whom we work, the partnerships we build, the research designs we employ, and even how we apply our findings. The social and professional lenses of the Tuskegee investigators enabled them to believe that the work they conducted was objective and inherently neutral. While most research is not purposefully predatory, a participant-centered approach may allow investigators access to other ways of thinking about their methodologic choices, thus avoiding similar victimization in any participant-driven research.

CONCLUSION

The Tuskegee Syphilis Study was designed to follow the natural progression of untreated syphilis, but the social and cultural footprint it left has further-reaching unforeseen implications. The disconnect between clinical research and racial/ethnic minority communities has been overly ascribed to this one historical abuse. Despite this and other breaches of morality and ethics in research, recent research has shown that African Americans in particular are still as willing to rise to the occasion of engaging in clinical research as other populations.[4-5,8,14] As researchers, and in light of this legacy, we are commissioned to handle their willingness with care. In addition to a resolve not to repeat the mistakes of the past, Tuskegee encourages us to consider how we establish and maintain presence within communities to create opportunities for access, reframes our thinking of communities as partners instead of solely as participants to ameliorate power and trust imbalances and persuades us to consider our individual and institutional responsibilities in increasing minority engagement with the research process.

Malika Roman Isler, PhD, MPH (research assistant professor of social medicine, UNC Chapel Hill School of Medicine), is a social scientist who has focused on socio-cultural constructions of health and models of community partnership in research. As the assistant director of the NC Translational and Clinical Sciences Institute Community Engagement Core, she facilitates community-based research infrastructures and capacity building to support community-academic partnerships in translational research. Her primary research focuses on community engagement in HIV prevention, HIV technology trials, population-based genomics initiatives, and access to HIV clinical trials.

Adebowale A. Odulana, MD, MPH (NRSA primary care research fellow at the Sheps Center for Health Services Research at UNC–Chapel Hill) is an internal medicine and pediatrics trained physician who has research interests in health disparities and pediatric obesity. He is currently working on research projects aimed at reducing minority health disparities through church-based participatory research and projects evaluating medical decision aids in relation to African American men.

Giselle Corbie-Smith, MD, MSc (professor in the Departments of Social Medicine and Medicine, UNC–Chapel Hill), is a clinician researcher who directs the Program on Health Disparities at the Sheps Center and the Community Engagement Core of the NC Translational and Clinical Sciences Institute. She is nationally recognized for her scholarly work on practical and ethical issues of involving communities of color in research and has served on numerous local, regional and national committees.

NOTES

1. National Institutes of Health. NIH Policy and Guidelines on The Inclusion of Women and Minorities as Subjects in Clinical Research 2001. http://grants.nih.gov /grants/funding/women_min/guidelines_amended_10_2001.htm.

2. Yancey, A. K., Ortega, A. N., and Kumanyika, S. K. Effective recruitment and retention of minority research participants. *Annu Rev Public Health.* 2006, 27:1–28.

3. Ford, J. G., Howerton, M. W., Lai, G. Y., et al. Barriers to recruiting underrepresented populations to cancer clinical trials: a systematic review. *Cancer.* Jan 15 2008, 112(2):228–242.

4. Katz, R. V., Green, B. L., Kressin, N. R., Claudio, C., Wang, M. Q., and Russell, S. L. Willingness of minorities to participate in biomedical studies: confirmatory

findings from a follow-up study using the Tuskegee Legacy Project Questionnaire. *J Natl Med Assoc.* Sep 2007, 99(9):1052–1060.

5. Katz, R. V., Kegeles, S. S., Kressin, N. R., et al. The Tuskegee Legacy Project: willingness of minorities to participate in biomedical research. *J Health Care Poor Underserved.* Nov 2006, 17(4):698–715.

6. McCallum, J. M., Arekere, D. M., Green, B. L., Katz, R. V., and Rivers, B. M. Awareness and knowledge of the U.S. Public Health Service syphilis study at Tuskegee: implications for biomedical research. *J Health Care Poor Underserved.* Nov 2006, 17(4):716–733.

7. Katz, R. V., Wang, M. Q., Green, B. L., et al. Participation in biomedical research studies and cancer screenings: perceptions of risks to minorities compared with whites. *Cancer Control.* Oct 2008, 15(4):344–351.

8. Wendler, D., Kington, R., Madans, J., et al. Are racial and ethnic minorities less willing to participate in health research? *PLoS Med.* Feb 2006, 3(2):e19.

9. Gross, D., and Fogg, L. Clinical trials in the 21st century: the case for participant-centered research. *Res Nurs Health.* Dec 2001, 24(6):530–539.

10. Thomas, S. B., and Quinn, S. C. The Tuskegee Syphilis Study, 1932 to 1972: implications for HIV education and AIDS risk education programs in the black community. *Am J Public Health.* Nov 1991, 81(11):1498–1505.

11. Trickett, E. J., and Espino, S. L. Collaboration and social inquiry: multiple meanings of a construct and its role in creating useful and valid knowledge. *Am J Community Psychol.* Sep 2004, 34(1–2):1–69.

12. CDC/ATSDR Committee on Community Engagement (U.S.); Centers for Disease Control and Prevention (U.S.), United States. Office of Public Health and Science. Principles of Community Engagement. *Part 1.* Atlanta, GA: Centers for Disease Control and Prevention; 1997: http://www.cdc.gov/phppo/pce/index.htm.

13. Shavers, V. L., Fagan, P., Lawrence, D., et al. Barriers to racial/ethnic minority application and competition for NIH research funding. *J Natl Med Assoc.* Aug 2005, 97(8):1063–1077.

14. Fouad, M. N., Corbie-Smith, G., Curb, D., et al. Special populations recruitment for the Women's Health Initiative: successes and limitations. *Control Clin Trials.* Aug 2004, 25(4):335–352.

Essay 10

Racial Conspiracy and Research

R. L'Heureux Lewis

The Tuskegee Syphilis Study holds a unique place in African American folklore and history simultaneously. To many, the United States Public Health Service (USPHS) Syphilis Study at Tuskegee, more commonly referred to as the Tuskegee Syphilis Study, is a hidden moment in history that reflects the exploitation of African Americans at the hands of government-sanctioned agents. Knowledge of the Tuskegee Syphilis Study remains fairly uneven, which makes its importance difficult to measure when looking at the relationship of African Americans to social and biomedical research. In this essay, I argue the Tuskegee Syphilis Study is a meaningful, yet not definitive, contributor to a generally strained relationship between African American communities and research. Lessons from, and limitations of, the Tuskegee Legacy Project (TLP), which produced seven key published papers of findings on racial differences on the willingness to participate in biomedical research and its relationship to the Tuskegee Syphilis Study (see Appendix B) as based upon two telephone surveys of adults in seven U.S. cities, can serve to elucidate how race matters in research conducted in the post–Civil Rights era.

EXPOSURE TO TUSKEGEE

I remember as a boy the first time I heard of the Tuskegee Experiment, as it was colloquially referred to in the communities where I was raised, I thought, "How could they do that to us?" I began to read more and the question morphed into, "Why should I have expected anything else since we were enslaved and experimented on for centuries?" The change in my question hinged not because of what I factually knew of the Tuskegee Syphilis Study; rather the question evolved because I began to understand there was a long-standing tradition of exploitation and endangerment of people of African descent.

I remember growing up and hearing of the Tuskegee Syphilis Study and being in utter shock. As I was told about the injection of African American men (this was not the only inaccuracy in the retelling) I was concerned that there was a world of information about the experiences of people of African descent of which I was unaware. Having a family that hails from Alabama, the story of the men with "bad blood" eventually moved from shock to anger and then became a piece of the race relations puzzle in the United States. I retell my experience with exposure to the Tuskegee Syphilis Study because it may be similar to many other African Americans' stories of encounter. To understand the potential meanings of the Tuskegee Syphilis Study we must unpack how its presence is transferred, how it is processed, and why it retains hold in some pockets of the African American community.

Exposure to the Tuskegee Syphilis Study does not necessarily mean that one will take a conspiratorial viewpoint; instead, most who are exposed likely encounter a crossroads. For some, Tuskegee is taken as an isolated and a sad moment in history. One could easily see this being the case among white Americans or people of color who doubt the sustained ill intent of the government. On the other hand, the Tuskegee Syphilis Study may be a lynchpin in theories of conspiracy against black Americans. This crossroads between isolated incident and conspiracy is one that all must negotiate. Ultimately, many will end up between both paths trying to make sense of the shortened life chances, the failed government interventions, and restricted opportunities of African Americans. One does not have to believe in conspiracy to hold a healthy skepticism toward "outsiders'" intentions for the African American community. Years after my discovery of the Tuskegee Syphilis Study and further reading, my outlook continued to shift until I took the perspective that at any given moment the African American community may be under threat. Even with this hanging reality, African Americans must negotiate social opportunities and hazards as they always exist. Because it is difficult to sidestep bad intentions, I did not stress complete disengagement from "outsiders," but I settled on cautious and selective engagement. Researchers are commonly thought of as outsiders to ethnic communities, in part, given the strained history where unethical treatment was normative.

RUMORS AND RACE

As I referenced earlier, when I first learned of the Tuskegee Syphilis Study I was told that the men were injected with syphilis by the US government. This idea remained as I learned more information about the medical and social mistreatment of African Americans that began when Africans arrived in captivity to the Americas and continued up through the Tuskegee Syphilis Study and beyond.[1,2] I found myself wondering, "What else could be happening right now, that I do not know about?" I have heard utterances in barbershops and family gatherings that a number of contemporary Tuskegee-like experiments were occurring. These "conspiracies" were justified by pointing to the disproportionately high rates of HIV/AIDS and other diseases within the black community. Given their lack of substantiation, I took them to be rumors, but these types of rumors exist and flourish for a reason among black communities.

Patricia Turner argued that contemporary African American conspiracies are a type of folklore that has its roots in the maltreatment of black populations that began with contact between Europeans and Africans.[3] In the 1980s and 1990s Turner collected narratives within the African American community that focused on covert attempts to exploit the black population, for example, rumors that the Ku Klux Klan secretly owned corporations with goals of black sterilization. She found that often these rumors were driven by past events where the labor, health, or the general livelihood of people of African descent was exploited. These rumors, while common in many Black communities, were less frequently known in white communities. This type of information asymmetry allowed for rumors to flourish and sentiments of skepticism to proliferate. The stream of exploitation of black people paints a grim portrait of African-European relations given the transatlantic slave trade, chattel slavery, sharecropping, Jim Crow, etc. This serves to animate suspicions that there are ongoing attempts to exploit black people or in extreme cases, exterminate black people. Turner argues, regardless of the viability of these race-related rumors, there is a rational explanation for their proliferation and maintenance that is often overlooked in studies of the African American community.

John Jackson argues that the post–Civil Rights era—the time after the passage of civil rights legislation when overt racism is less common—has bred racial paranoia for blacks and whites alike.[4,5] Jackson says, "The concept of racial paranoia, however, stresses the fears I've been talking about, fears people harbor about other groups potentially hating or mistreating them, gaining a leg up at their expense. Racial paranoia is racism's flipside . . .

(pg. 4)."[5] This fear of being "one-upped" can be seen in contemporary discussions on both sides of the black-white racial divide. With television commentators like Glenn Beck blaring that President Barack Obama is a closeted Muslim and socialist who hates whites, the fears of black political power serve to dislodge the comfort of many white Americans. On the other hand, the decreases in overt racist expressions have led to the adages in the black community like "racism didn't die, they don't wear Klan robes any more, they wear judge's robes." The aforementioned quote highlights the ways the current criminal justice system has led to the disproportionate incarceration of blacks and Latinos.[6] A look at the racial landscape reveals that blacks remain disproportionately poor, incarcerated, unhealthy, and lodged in low-quality neighborhoods with failing schools. These conditions provide ample reason to believe that something beyond individual effort is driving the "failure" of the black community. The deep scars left from centuries of racism make it understandable that blacks may view the actions of government as synonymous with the interests of whites, even when their intentions may not be.

The telling of the Tuskegee Syphilis Study as including the injection of syphilis is common because the event is verifiable but the details are not as easily accessible. As a result, verification of the occurrence leads to a slippery slope of acceptances that may not conform to actual historical events. When I was exposed to the Tuskegee Syphilis Study, with bad information, I was also exposed to the idea that it was a conspiracy with the goal of killing black men. Jackson points out, "[the] more extreme version of the general racial and cultural paranoia that threads itself through much of African American public discourse and highlights the profound inadequacies of sight—a seeing that demands believing and disbelieving at the same time. (pg. 94)"[4] In this constellation, perfect information is not necessary; partial information animates paranoia.

Given that accurate knowledge of the Tuskegee Syphilis Study is uncommon and overall knowledge of Tuskegee is limited, it is doubtful that the Tuskegee Syphilis Study affects widespread disengagement of research. Instead, a general racial paranoia, in part informed by Tuskegee, influences black disengagement. For some, the link in the chain of exploitation of black people in the Americas is strong and may influence engagement in research. For those, knowledge of the Tuskegee Syphilis Study may cause them to opt out of the sample when contacted for any survey, including the Tuskegee Legacy Project's two surveys in 2000 and 2003. Opting out of research is one of the great concerns that the legacy of the Tuskegee Syphilis Study carries, hence the Tuskegee Legacy Project may not have captured those with the most adversarial relationships to research.

RESPONSE AND OMISSION

The Tuskegee Legacy Project (TLP) papers contribute significantly to the literature on research, culture and participation. All seven papers draw a similar conclusion, that African Americans are more likely to have heard of the Tuskegee experiment, are not likely to recall specifics, and this knowledge and nonknowledge are not linked to willingness to participate or fear of being a guinea pig in medical research. In a number of the studies, Katz et al. (see list of TLP articles in Appendix B) find that knowledge of the Tuskegee Syphilis Study varies along racial lines and knowledge is strongest among those closest to the epicenter of Tuskegee. Much like an earthquake, information and knowledge about the Tuskegee Syphilis Study are strongest near the source and less so on the periphery. The ripple was likely carried for many years orally and in recent years via film and books. These ripples can influence also who is captured within a research sample, and who is not.

The seven TLP reports authoritatively paint a picture that the Tuskegee Syphilis Study has little influence on the participation of blacks or other communities in biomedical research. The strengths of the TLP are in the studies' empirics, but the weaknesses are in the methodology. The use of telephone survey is common practice among survey methodologies, but phone surveys of vulnerable populations also raise a number of concerns. Gurin, Hatchett and Jackson in their discussion of the National Black Election Study detailed the additional steps that were necessary to ensure a representative black population when using phone surveys.[7] Undercoverage and nonresponse are two key issues that have troubled gathering representative telephone surveys among black Americans.

Undercoverage refers to the concern that the sampling frame has not covered certain segments of a population. Typically, black and low-income populations fail to be adequately captured. Because traditional phone random digit dialing is based on achieving a statistically representative sample, this type of coverage is often insufficient in developing a robust portrait of black Americans. Katz et al. (see TLP article in Appendix B) have done a commendable job in gathering a large number of blacks, but the representativeness of these black respondents remains in question. Gurin et al. argue that stratifying by metropolitan statistical areas is essential to ensuring that studies are not drawing from black populations of a particular type.[8] Often samples are not drawn with a particular consciousness of residential patterns and tend to sample easily accessible portions of vulnerable populations rather than representative respondents. In the case of city-based surveys, sampling across census tracts or with consideration of residential segregation would be essential to capturing adequate vulnerable populations. Despite their request of twenty years ago, this is seldom done because sampling frames are traditionally based on the distribution of whites, rather than blacks (for more discussion on black-centered sampling frames please see Jackson, Neighbors, Nesse, Trierweiler, and Torres).[9] This is commonly the case with contracted telephone survey companies.

Undercoverage is meaningful because many low-income families, particularly the black poor, are not surveyed due to lack of phone lines. The Pew Center's report "What's Missing from National RDD surveys? The growing problem of cell-phone only" finds that young adults are particularly undercovered in surveys given the increasing numbers of people who lack a landline but use cell phones only.[10] A follow-up survey in 2010 found that cell-phone-only use was also more common among racial minority communities.[11] This issue of undercoverage remains in the era of cell phone technology in part because time spent on calls is often attached to direct fees (e.g. monthly minutes). With fewer economic resources, greater reliance on mobile technology and a lengthy survey, many segments of the black population may have been overlooked.

Nonresponse likely represents another significant issue with the TLP. The central question becomes, are the populations that are willing to partake in research different than those who refuse to participate? The TLP Questionnaire was a 60-item survey instrument that averaged 25 minutes to complete. While not the longest survey, it remains a significant time commitment. It is logical to think that the person who agrees to participate in a research study is already more likely to view research favorably than those who refuse to participate. Even if they are not more favorable toward research, they may be more familiar with research and thus more comfortable. Second, those who decide to participate in research may be more likely to endorse participating in research than those who have an adversarial or uninterested relationship to research and opted out of the phone survey. This chain of association is likely given those who opt to complete a 60-question survey are already demonstrating a proclivity for participation in research. It would only be logical that those who had a disinterest in research or serious concerns about the invasion of privacy and/or their physical bodies would opt out of the survey to begin with.

In my experience, the willingness to engage in research is first identified at the point of contact. If the phone survey used a screener question to begin with that asked for race, age, income and other key demographics, knowing who answered that screener and then opted out would be most helpful. A secondary, but less powerful, option would be knowing response rates by race and class and seeing if there is variation in captured respondents to help identify the types of selection into the sample. Neither of these two types of data were obtained in the TLP surveys. Whether in quantitative or qualitative research, the task of capturing respondents of color has proven difficult for researchers across the color and class line. In my own research, being an African American researcher has marginally aided in securing more research subjects. Even when respondents from vulnerable populations have responded to my research queries and known I was African American, they have opted out of participating at rates that were disproportionate to white respondents. This suggests that understanding the gaps between abstract agreement to participation and actual participation are greater than often considered.

BELIEFS VS. BEHAVIOR

The TLP Questionnaire directly asks respondents to identify research-related behaviors in which they would or world not engage. While they found little evidence for difference in endorsement of willingness to participate, I am skeptical that this reflects actual respondents' behaviors. Schuman, Steeh, Bobo and Krysan argue that surveys capture attitudes (also called beliefs by some) and that attitudes only constitute part of behaviors.[12] There is often a lack of alignment between attitudes and behaviors regarding sensitive subjects and behaviors. Given that biomedical research consistently suffers from undercoverage among communities of color and other segments of the population, those participating in the survey may be answering in the abstract or in a socially desirable fashion. This is not to suggest attitudinal measures have no place; rather, it is to suggest that they must be placed in context and not assumed to be a perfect reflection of behavior.

What may be necessary to gain participation may be entirely different than getting one to endorse a positive attitude toward research. Given the extensive literature on the use of incentives to attract "vulnerable populations" I am led to believe that the TLP's findings confirm that the Tuskegee Syphilis Study has little import on the abstract idea of participation among those who already hold a favorable relationship to research.[13] However, when posed with the potential of injection by IV or actually taking experimental medicine, abstract sentiments of agreement will likely be challenged. Given that many biomedical research projects provide incentives and still find lower participation among vulnerable populations, there appear to be factors that lie between abstractly agreeing to research participation and engaging as a research participant.

TUSKEGEE SYPHILIS STUDY'S LEGACY WITHIN RACIAL PARANOIA

Understanding the reasons behind the participation (or lack thereof) of black communities in research is a difficult task. The Tuskegee Legacy Project has contributed notably to our understanding about the role of events such as the Tuskegee Syphilis Study, but can only get us partly "out of the woods" in dilemmas of research engagement with vulnerable populations. In this essay, I have identified multiple issues that likely affect the participation of African Americans in research. The role of racial conspiracy will continue to affect African Americans as we remember and imagine the past while experiencing the present. The TLP's study findings can allay some fears of widescale direct contamination of the Tuskegee Syphilis Study, but it cannot serve to debase concerns of exploitation of communities of color in relation to research.

The toxins of the racial past are passed informally and can serve to supplant ethically conducted research. Contextualizing past atrocities, such as providing accurate information about the Tuskegee Syphilis Study, is still not enough given the current environment of racial paranoia. With more information like the Henrietta Lacks story [14] and the sterilization of Puerto Rican women [15] coming forward about communities of color more fodder for concern is piling. It is the responsibility of researchers and the biomedical community to understand the roots of these discomforts and creatively engage communities of color ethically. In social science research there has been an increased emphasis on community-based participatory research in which communities and researchers are partners in developing and executing research.[16] While this form of work has its own sets of issues, the potential for extension into varying forms of research may be valuable. The next decade poses a challenge to our methodologies and strategies of engagement as researchers. The past is undeniably tied to the present, but we must figure out where those attachments lie so that new ethically grounded and representative research can be undertaken.

R. L'Heureux Lewis, PhD (assistant professor, Department of Sociology and Black Studies Program, City University of New York–CUNY), is a sociologist who focuses on issues of race and ethnicity. His work concentrates on African American education, health, and gender relations. His major line of research explores how inequality is structured and how policy responses can reduce these inequalities. He is the author of the forthcoming book Inequality in the Promised Land: New Dilemmas in Race, Education and Opportunity. *He was selected as a Ford Foundation Diversity Fellow and an American Sociological Association Mental Health Minority Fellow.*

NOTES

1. Washington, H. (2008). *Medical apartheid: The dark history of medical experimentation on black americans from colonial times to the present.* New York: Knopf Doubleday Publishing Group.

2. A number of these incidents were passed along orally and I did not see written confirmation of them or similar acts until Harriet Washington published *Medical Apartheid* in 2007.

3. Turner, P. (1994). *I heard it through the grapevine: Rumor in African-American culture.* California: University of California Press.

4. Jackson, J. J. (2004). *Real black adventures in racial sincerity.* Chicago: University of Chicago Press.

5. Jackson, J. J. (2008). *Racial paranoia: The unintended consequences of political correctness.* New York: Basic Civitas Books.

6. Alexander, M. (2010). *The new Jim Crow: Mass incarceration in the age of colorblindness.* New York; Jackson, Tenn.: New Press; Distributed by Perseus Distribution.

7. Gurin, P., Hatchett, S., & Jackson, J. (1989). *Hope and independence: Blacks' response to electoral and party politics.* New York: The Russell Sage Foundation.

8. While Gurin and Jackson's discussion is based on national data, their points stand when sampling cities given levels of residential segregation.

9. Jackson, J., Neighbors, H., Nesse, R., Trierweiler, S., Torres, M., (2004). Methodological innovations in the national survey of American life. *International Journal of Methods in Psychiatric Research* 13(4), 289–298.

10. Keeter, S., Kennedy, C., Clark, A., Tompson, T., & Mokrzycki, M. (2007). *What's missing from national RDD surveys? The impact of the growing cell-only population.* Pew Research Center for the People & the Press.

11. Christian, L., Keeter, S., Purcell, K., & Smith, A. (2010). *Assessing the cell phone challenge* Pew Internet & American Life Project.

12. Schuman, H., Steeh, C., Bobo, L., & Krysan, M. (1997). *Racial attitudes in America: Trends and interpretations* (Revised Edition). Cambridge, MA: Harvard University Press.

13. Yancey, A., Ortega, A., & Kumanyika, S. (2006). Effective recruitment and retention of minority research participants. *Annual Review of Public Health* 27, 1–28.

14. Skloot, R. (2010). *The immortal life of Henrietta Lacks.* New York: Crown Publishing.

15. Lopez, I. (2008). *Matters of choice: Puerto Rican women's struggle for reproductive freedom.* New Jersey: Rutgers University.

16. Minkler, M. (2005). Community based research partnerships: Challenges and opportunities. *Journal of Urban Health,* (83), 3–12.

Essay 11

African Americans and the Broader Legacy of Experience with the American Health Care Community

Parasites, Locusts, and Scavengers

Harold L. Aubrey

The historical and contemporary collective experiences of African Americans within the health care establishment in the United States of America are a multi-structural complex set of dynamic activities. Among African Americans, the legacy of the Tuskegee Syphilis Study represents a "mere poster child" of literally thousands of negative experiences etched in the memory of African Americans across generations and socioeconomic classes. Moreover, the unabated predominance of negative experiences with the American health care community continues to frame the perceptions of African Americans to this day.

The Tuskegee Syphilis Study is merely a widely acknowledged "face" representing literally thousands of such medical research studies that have involved African Americans with real and perceived negative experiences. The vast majority of such studies have left participants and the larger African American community with negative perceptions. Prevailing historical records along with more contemporary health care experiences simply reinforce real and perceived negative perceptions of African Americans regarding the American health care community.

The legacy of the Tuskegee Syphilis Study is not an entity unto itself. It is but one of the multitude of medals connected by a continuous chain of medals representing the collective health care experiences of African Americans. Those medals on that chain have been shaped in multiple designs and sizes. Medals representing the Tuskegee Syphilis Study are very large. This description of an imaginary chain of medals is proffered as a functional concept to view the contextual legacy of a much larger landscape.

Additionally, the title of this essay uses a set of terms that provide more lucid context for the players in the saga of observations in the broader legacy of the African American experience with the American health care community. Webster defines a parasite as a person who lives at the expense of another or others without making any useful contribution or return. Locusts are defined by Webster as any of various large grasshoppers; specifically, a migratory grasshopper often traveling in great swarms and destroying nearly all vegetation in areas visited. Scavengers are defined as animals, such as birds or insects, that feed on dead or decaying matter.

Further, a more structural analysis of the legacy of the Tuskegee Syphilis Study must provide some attention to its chronological context and attention to prevailing environmental forces in key developmental periods. Therefore, I have selectively identified some of those key forces which shaped science and the societal environment that facilitated the Tuskegee Syphilis Study. Some observations of the former's connection to the legacy of the Tuskegee Syphilis Study are discussed. A novel mathematical model, Aubrey's Triple E Triangular Model of Outcome Probabilities, is used to identify threads of similarity across observations in a more structured manner similar to the chain and medals metaphor.[1]

AUBREY'S TRIPLE E TRIANGULAR MODEL OF OUTCOME PROBABILITIES

Aubrey's Triple E Triangular Model of Outcome Probabilities is an in-development framework that is designed to support a structural analysis of phenomena in which multiple sets of variables are reduced to three composite variables. The Triple Es are the composite variables: Educational Achievement, Economic Condition and Exploitation Degree. The first two composite variables provide inputs and outputs continuously to jointly produce a third sub-index whose value is a determinant of the degree of exploitation of the individual or group. Regarding this essay, Aubrey's Triple E Triangular Model of Outcome Probabilities' quantitative method of analysis is illustrative of the interplay and resultant summation by the three key composite variables.[1]

Educational achievement and economic condition are composite independent predictor covariates. Exploitation degree (or degree of exploitation) is a composite dependent outcome variable. The basic computational formula is: $A^2 \pm B^2 = C$ (Education Achievement Value $\pm$ Economic Condition Value = Exploitation Degree). Variables in the basic equation are all composed of an infinite number of multiple sub-categorical variables which span four quartile levels. The computational process is designed to quantify observational data and facilitate interpretation of summary results.

Individuals or groups with lower educational achievement values generally experience lower values in relation to economic condition. Consequently, those individuals or groups will generally experience greater degrees of exploitation in their lives. Given that observation, the mean value indicates that the more advantaged players use their position to exploit less advantaged individuals or groups in a given society. The development of modern inferential statistics was a driver of modern scientific research and the parallel development of the eugenics movement will be used to illustrate how science and the social environment operate to encourage exploitation of the disadvantaged by the advantaged. That backdrop broadly set the stage for the commencement of the Tuskegee Syphilis Study.

THE DAWN OF MODERN INFERENTIAL STATISTICS AND LINKS TO THE BIRTH OF EUGENICS

The genesis of the modern era in inferential statistics began with Francis Galton's invention of regression analysis in the early 1880s. Many view the development of regression analysis as a major milestone in the evolution of modern inferential statistics. The core of regression analysis is rooted in Adrien-Marie Legendre's method of least square, but Galton is credited as the father of regression analysis.[12] Galton's work in statistics as well as the work of his protégés and their contemporaries provided major pillars on which the foundation of modern statistical inference still rests. Particularly noteworthy among his protégés were Karl Pearson, George Yule and Francis Edgeworth.[13]

Conceptual and theoretical developments led to applications in experimental studies and other research problems in every area of scientific research. Concepts such as variation, natural selection, randomization and modern sampling techniques were developed by Galton and his protégés. Invention of those statistical procedures was the beginning of the modern development of classes of statistical methods. They remain hallmarks of scientific research studies. Of course, young Ronald Fisher among others was a major player. [5,6,10]

Undoubtedly, Galton's key protégé was Pearson. Pearson is viewed as Galton's statistical heir apparent. During his lifetime, Pearson wrote significant volumes of research papers, books, etc. with nineteen major papers considered as classics. In addition to his statistical pursuits, Pearson pursued the development and codification of eugenics aggressively. He was not alone in having mixed interests in both inferential statistics and eugenics. Seward

Wright is another major figure in the development of modern inferential statistics. He is considered a major contributor to the development of theoretical population genetics and inventor of the inbreeding coefficient and gene frequencies, among other modern scientific developments.[3,4]

Several of the major players in the development of the modern inferential statistics that still drives modern scientific research (particularly modern medical research) were also active movers and shakers in the eugenics movement. Clearly, works of these individuals in statistics and eugenics provided "scientific validation" for the thinking that propelled the eugenics movement. Ultimately, this contributed to acceptance and the societal environment that launched the Tuskegee Syphilis Study and other such studies in the name of "science."

THE RISE OF THE EUGENICS MOVEMENT IN AMERICA

Charles Davenport is the major American figure having a leading role in promoting the establishment of eugenics as a major social and public policy in U.S. After 1900, Galton began to experience a decline in his health leading to his death in 1911. He had already started transference of his work to his protégé Pearson, whose professional interests included eugenics. During this same period, Davenport was aggressively institutionalizing the eugenics movement by guiding it from a scientific idea to a worldwide movement that many nations implemented.

The existence of eugenics as a public policy entity created a macro environment in the American scientific research community where specific categories of American citizens were marginalized and considered ideal candidates for use as subjects in scientific studies. Using Aubrey's Triple E Triangular Model, specific categories of American citizens that were identified as potential research subjects could be described as members of the group with the lowest index of educational achievement and economic conditional probabilities. Clearly, the marginalized and near-marginalized American citizenry were prime targets for recruitment into studies and eventual exploitation. These marginalized and near-marginalized American citizens were generally:

1. Members of the lowest classes of the educational achievement
2. The lowest classes of the economically disadvantaged in society.

After the stock market crash of 1929, those most educationally and economically marginalized and near marginal citizenry were great targets for social and political exploitation. Again, that prevailing social, political and economic environment greatly facilitated the type of thinking that undergirded decisions regarding study protocol development for the Tuskegee Syphilis Study and other such studies.

THE EUGENICS MOVEMENT AND MEDICAL EXPERIMENTS IN NAZI GERMANY

While the Tuskegee Syphilis Study was underway in America and the American eugenics movement was rising to a zenith, the eugenics movement in Nazi Germany had moved to an unprecedented level of horror. The most heinous systematic human experimentation in the name of medical research was descending to a new depth unseen in human history.

After World War II, Karl Brandt and twenty-two other Nazis were tried and convicted at Nuremberg, Germany, for crimes against humanity. That trial is commonly referred as the "Doctors' Trial." One direct legacy of the Nuremberg Trials was a document submitted to the Nuremberg Council for War Crimes that sought to define legitimate medical research. Originally, the document contained six points and four additional points were added later. The revised document containing ten points became known as the Nuremberg Code. This was the start of a major attempt to legally ban inhumane human experimentation in any kind of research.[9]

Unfortunately, that development has had little impact on the widespread views of the advantaged relative to their more disadvantaged cohorts. Little has changed in the ebb and flow of social thought irrespective of national locality. Generally, the marginal and near-marginal citizenry of different societies are still viewed as insignificant.

Long before the end of World War II and the adoption of the Nuremberg Code, an effective treatment for syphilis had been discovered. Because they were not viewed as worthy of the most basic human consideration, the subjects of the Tuskegee Syphilis Study were denied that treatment. Consequently, the United States Public Health Service continued the exploitation of the African American male subjects of the Tuskegee Syphilis Study. The continuance of systematic benign neglect of those human subjects was a violation of the Nuremberg Code.

THE CONCEPTUAL ENVIRONMENT OF THE TUSKEGEE SYPHILIS STUDY AND AIDS PANDEMIC

The Tuskegee Syphilis Study was designed and implemented in the early 1930s because of a pressing public health need to find an effective treatment for syphilis. However, major advances in modern medical research methodologies were widely known. Those advances included clinical trial protocol development, the conduct of studies, human subject selection, use of results, etc. The U.S. Public Health Service was not operating in isolation from those advances. But decisions that were made regarding the Tuskegee study supported grossly inhuman treatment of study subjects. These decisions were deeply reflective of the prevailing social and political climate that was poisoned with a eugenics mind-set.

African American male subjects of the Tuskegee Syphilis Study had not experienced any serious education to speak of and were desperately poor. Consequently, they were marginalized and severely exploited. This observation is consistent with the basic premise of Aubrey's Triple E Triangular Model.

Negative perceptions of the American health care community have been further reinforced by the spread of the AIDS pandemic. Negative opinions and rumors concerning the origin and continued scourge of the AIDS virus have continued to light wildfires in African American communities all across America. Perceptions remain that this pandemic was developed to eliminate African Americans. Whether there is any truth to those perceptions or not, negative perceptions still persist.

More recently, information concerning the origin and development of HeLa cells have been widely reported.[7] George Otto Gey extracted a sample of cancer extracted from the cervix of Henrietta Lacks. That extraction has become an immortalized human cell line. This occurred at the Johns Hopkins University Hospital in 1951. No one ever sought permission to study Ms. Lacks's cells. Finally, her family was told of this act more than twenty years after it occurred. Incidentally, the design of the Tuskegee study was developed by a Johns Hopkins scientist.[2]

While little was written about this case until approximately a decade ago, a large body of material exists on the story of HeLa cells. As a consequence, another "poster child" was born. Public sentiment amongst African Americans is negative. The primary opinion is that the medical research establishment exploited Ms. Lacks and her survivors.[11]

A VIEW FROM THE BRIDGE

Throughout the course of human history, there have been events of subterfuge, tragedy, triumph, and defeat. Unfortunately, the landscape of that same history is plastered with an abundance of evidence pointing to a consistent lack of a "level playing field." The lack of a level playing field has persisted. In all areas of human existence, the aforementioned observation has been consistently woven into the fabric of human experiences. The continuous evolving tapestry of human experiences can be characterized, interpreted, and summarized in as many ways as scholarly thought can imagine. A multitude of explanations are possible principally because of the infinite number of resultant by-products of human interaction within the integral complexity of nano-functional behavioral structures.

If recorded human history is prologue, then some of the more fundamental characteristics of human existence and experience now, in the foreseeable future, and in the long-term future are not likely to change. In essence, the more things change the more they stay the same. One quartile of humanity in any society functions as though they have inherited a license to abuse the remaining three quartiles without an iota of moral fiber or ethical obligation. Unfortunately, the record of human history is replete with evidence of the aforementioned notion. It is an ugly legacy that has been passed from one generation to another in every society known to humanity.

The eminent Swedish sociologist Gunnar Myrdal strongly criticized the bias in existing empirical "research" literature. Myrdal devoted considerable attention to this problem in his classic study, *An American Dilemma: the Negro Problem and Modern Democracy.* In his review of research on the American Negro problem, he stated that:

> The underlying psychology of bias in science is simple. Every individual student is himself more or less entangled, both as a private person and as a responsible citizen, in a web of conflicting variations. Like a layman, through probably to a lesser extent, the scientist becomes influenced by the need for rationalizations. The same is true of every executive responsible for other people's research and of the popular and scientific public which the scholar performs, and whose reactions he must respect. Against, the most honest determination to be open-minded on the part of all concerned and primarily on the part of the scientists themselves, the need for rationalization will tend to influence the objects chosen for research, the selection of relevant data, the recording of observations, the theoretical and practical inferences drawn and the manner of presentation of results.

Myrdal's pointed observations are as true today as they were when the classic study was published nearly a half century ago.[8]

The scientific community in America remains a reflection of legacy and inheritance. The statistical evidence suggests that observation of reality is blinded by many unspoken truths, denials, contradictions, and excuses. A longitudinal analysis of existing historical and contemporary statistical data will simply provide an unbroken pattern of consistent results, based more on scientists' rationalizations than upon scientific reasoning.

The key factor of cultural dynamics continues to be a major pitfall in the research literature when African Americans are subjects of that research. Far too many researchers are guilty of viewing the culture of African American subjects as a minor distraction or a static phenomenon. In addition, those same researchers view African Americans as a "monolithic collection of people." Little evidence of comprehension of African American cultural history exists among contemporary scientific researchers. As a consequence, major flaws in research design, data collection, and interpretation are as routine as was observed by Myrdal in his day.

During the last decade, some significant research studies have been published concerning health disparities. African Americans have been key subjects of those studies. However, critical examinations of the more significant studies indicate that some of the same historical flaws in design, data collection, and interpretation are still prevalent. A good example is the attempts to determine the extent to which African Americans will participate in clinical trials. Too often the focus is on the influence of the Tuskegee Syphilis Study and many other such studies are ignored.

Although published studies that have sought to address the aforementioned issue are generally sound, a closer review reveals design flaws regarding significant African American cultural factors. In particular, there are some critical cultural questions that must be critically examined in the pre–design protocol development phase. Some of those questions are:

- How much is known about the Tuskegee Syphilis Study across generations of African Americans?
- What is the African American cultural history literacy level across generations of African Americans?
- What is the quality of the health care experience among African Americans across generations of African Americans?
- What is the extent of intra-group geographical differences among African Americans regarding health care experiences?
- What is the extent of intra-group socioeconomic differences among African Americans in respect to geographical locale regarding health care experience?

Unfortunately, as long as there is a paucity of experts of African American descent among the pool of scientific researchers in general and biomedical researchers in particular, little change will occur. Additionally, significant negative perceptions of medical research in particular and research in general will continue to persist among African Americans.

Harold L. Aubrey, MS, MURP, EdD (partner, Calstar Investments, LLC) is an applied statistician. In the last 20 years, he has served as a consultant, co-author or author of more than 150 research, evaluation, and planning reports. His primary specialty is the application of advanced statistical methods in the design of experimental and nonexperimental research in education, public health, social sciences, and behavioral sciences. While serving as a higher education administrator (chair, director, assistant dean, dean, assistant vice president, and acting provost) and professor, he has been a chair or committee member of 21 doctoral dissertations.

NOTES

1. Aubrey, H. (2010). Aubrey's Triple E Triangular Model of Outcome Probabilities, Development of a Structural Analytical Model for Longitudinal Research (work in progress) Lincoln University (PA).

2. Brown, R., and J. Henderson (1983). "The Mass Production and Distribution of HeLa Cells at Tuskegee Institute, 1953–1955." *Journal of History Med Allied Science* 38 (4):415–43.

3. Crow, J., and W. Dove (1987). "Sewall Wright and Physiological Genetics." *Genetics* 115 (1): 1–2.

4. Crow, J. F. (1988). "Sewall Wright (1889–1988)." *Genetics* 119 (1): 1–4.

5. Edwards, A. (2005). "R. A. Fisher, Statistical Methods for Research Workers, 1925." In I. Grattan-Guinness (ed.), *Landmark Writings in Western Mathematics: Case Studies, 1640–1940*, Amsterdam: Elsevier.

6. Fisher, R. (1918). "The Correlation Between Relatives on the Supposition of Mendelian Inheritance." *Transactions Royal Society of Edinburgh* 52: 399–433.

7. Masters, J. (2002). "HeLa Cells 50 Years On: The Good, the Bad and the Ugly." *Nature Reviews Cancer* 2 (4): 315–19.

8. Myrdal, G. (1962). *An American Dilemma: The Negro Problem and Modern Democracy.* New York: Harper & Row, Publishers, 1035–1036

9. Nelkin, D., and M. Michaels (1998). "Biological Categories and Border Controls: The Revival of Eugenics in Anti-Immigration Rhetoric." *International Journal of Sociology and Social Research*, 18: 35–64.

10. Neyman, J., and Pearson, E. (1933). "On the Problem of the Most Efficient Tests of Statistical Hypothesis." *Philosophical Transactions of the Royal Society of London*, Series A: 231, 289–337.

11. Skloot, R. (2010). *The Immortal Life of Henrietta Lacks.* New York City: Random House.

12. Smith, D. (1959). *A Source Book in Mathematics Vol. II.* New York: McGraw-Hill (1929) and Dover (1959): 576–579.

13. Stanton, J. (2001): "Galton, Pearson, and the Peas: A Brief History of Linear Regression for Statistics Instructors." *Journal of Statistics Education*, 9 (3).

Essay 12

The USPHS Syphilis Study at Tuskegee

Rethinking the Horizons of Beneficence

Riggins R. Earl Jr.

The shared value assumption, based on the Hippocratic Oath, is that medical researchers and practitioners in the name of beneficence are working for the common good of the patient. By so doing, such professionals are contributing to the common good of society. This taken-for-granted value assumption is derived from the classical philosophical belief that the *means* for achieving the common good must be virtuous. Bioethicist Robert Veatch, acknowledging the potential conflict between human actions and motives, makes an important contrasting definitive distinction between *benevolence* and *beneficence*:

> Benevolence is a virtue of willing to do good. Beneficence is a principle of actions, the principle of actually acting in such a way that good consequences result. One can of course will the good (show the virtue of benevolence) but end up not doing the good (being beneficent). One can also be malevolent, but nevertheless beneficent. (This person would not be of good will, but would nevertheless act in such a way that good results are produced, perhaps because the malevolent one has calculated that it is in his or her self-interest to produce the good consequences).[1]

The crux of the problem here is that most bioethicists ignore the relationship of the beneficence narratives[2] in their discourses on the society's larger malevolent/benevolent narratives of race, class and gender. That is to say, bioethicists, reluctant to expand their social horizons, have been mainly concerned about choosing the right action and less with structures and

117

patterns of meaning.[3] Consequently bioethicists' discourses of beneficence, too often, are limited to the medical context of doing the right thing individually. For this reason they run the danger of adhering to a limited, if not subverted, version of beneficence even in the clinical context. For instance, Pellegrino and Thomasma, in their book *The Patient's Good: The Restoration of Beneficence in Health Care,*[4] fail to factor race, class, and gender into their otherwise rigorous ethical analysis. This limited approach, which illustrates the claim, runs the danger of isolating bioethicists in their intellectual ghettos (e.g., hospitals and the university); leaving them to revel in their own narrowly crafted discursive presuppositions and conclusions about the patients' good. It separates them from the larger lived world of the different narrative voices[5] of their patients, whose experiences are determined by race, class, and gender. Such voices, alienated and subverted though they may be, challenge those of the medical community to rethink often inherent ethical tensions between *willing the good* and *doing the good.* The bioethicist's challenge is to appreciate critically the tension between malevolent, benevolent and beneficent narrative voices regarding questions of social justice. This must be done in light of the patients' good and vice versa. Contemporary bioethicists fail, in this way, to expand the moral horizons of their discourses, consequently failing to nuance ethical insights from the larger lived world.[6] In short, bioethicists fail to value different lived experiences, sometimes even their own.

The primary thesis here is that a socio-ethical[7] probing of the Tuskegee Syphilis Study, which is seriously lacking in the literature, is absolutely necessary. (No major ethical study has been done as of yet.) Surprisingly, black ethicists have practically ignored this area for investigation.[8] It is fundamentally necessary to challenge bioethicists, who are primarily white,[9] to rethink the hermeneutical limitations of their modern discourses of the application of beneficence. The Tuskegee Syphilis Study and its cultural determinants of race, class, and gender demand that we do this from a historical perspective, providing different angles of hermeneutical insight regarding beneficence.[10]

Different narrative voices of beneficence (in relationship to benevolence and malevolence) have shaped the historical ethos of America in general and the Tuskegee Syphilis Study context in particular. As certain voices indicate, the Study was about more than how untreated syphilis worked in the bodies of poor black men of the Alabama rural South. In the larger picture, it was about how the consequences of the disease affected the men, physically and morally, and their lived worlds of familial relationships.[11] This fact alone challenges bioethicists to broaden and deepen their socio-ethical analyses of the Tuskegee Study in particular and their bioethical discourses in general.

Here it will be shown how views of benevolence, which have their roots in the making of New England Puritanism[12] (Jonathan Edwards), Southern slavery,[13] and the Abolitionist Movement[14] (Samuel Hopkins) shaped America's meta-narratives. Skewed interpretations of benevolence and beneficence also produced and supported the makers and custodians of slavery and racial segregation in America[15] (segregationist literature). Practices of slavery and segregation, in the name of benevolence, and occasionally beneficence, produced the social and moral climate for the making of all the players, victimizers and victims, of the infamous syphilis study. Meanwhile, advocates of benevolence and justice produced the moral impetus for the abolition of slavery, the making of Tuskegee Institute and later University, and the desegregation of American society. The desegregation movement, in the name of love, power and justice, produced a more favorable moral and social climate for former President William Jefferson Clinton to make his Presidential Apology and for the public to receive it.

The remainder of this essay proposes to illuminate the thesis by probing ethically the following questions in light of the narrative voices (i.e., cultural determinants) of race, class, and gender: a) The ethical question of President Clinton's apology: an act of beneficence or benevolence? b) The ethical question of subverted beneficence and the researchers' and victims' undergirded lived worlds of pseudoscience, religion, benevolence, class, and race, and c) the question of the possible consequential good derivable from the infamous study.

THE ETHICAL QUESTION OF THE APOLOGY

Better than a decade ago President William Jefferson Clinton, in a White House ceremony, apologized to the black survivors of the federal government's infamous syphilis study.[16] Scholars have differed in their assessment as to whether Clinton's apology was an act of beneficence or benevolence?—i.e., an act of doing good or willing it in response to the tragedy. Some rightfully questioned the sincerity of the president's apology, suggesting that he was politically pandering to blacks. Constructively responding to critics of the apology, historian Susan Reverby notes, in all fairness to the president's intent that the apology was about racism:

> The president's rhetoric, as communication scholars noted a few years later, put radical injustice, "not medical ethics and abuse of power," at the center of the problem. Clinton's language made it clear that the apology was not just from

the PHS or the government. It was from the American people. The institute's role in the Study was made to be peripheral and the desire for racial reconciliation was made simpler. Science became value-free, as only racial politics, not something inherent in the way scientific ideas are constructed, became the cause of the Study and at the center of what went wrong. The apology thus became an apology for racism and not really about the role of medicine and science in the creation of beliefs about race.[17]

The more pressing ethical aspect of the apology, it seems, has to do with the president's demonstrable courage in facing the historical truth of the nation's injustice to blacks. Clinton demonstrated rare courage by apologizing, admitting that whites misconstrued the use of science to support false claims of racial superiority. The indisputable fact is that Clinton became the first president in the history of the nation to apologize to blacks for the nation's injustice to them. The apology itself provides a powerful symbolic white alternative narrative voice to white America's degrading narrative of blacks, beginning with the slave trade out of Africa.

Clinton's apology took place almost seventy years after the Tuskegee Syphilis Study began in Macon County, Alabama, under the auspices of the federal government.[18] To be sure, it took place in a more race-friendly political and moral social era than did the Study. A product himself of the same segregated South in which the Study was conducted, Clinton was the beneficiary of a more favorable climate of race relations. That favorable climate of race relations was the consequence of the Civil Rights Movement, which was led by the moral leadership of Martin L. King, Jr. and Malcolm X. Procedurally, Clinton's apology for the Study, it is safe to say, was the result of the challenging request made by the Tuskegee Legacy Committee,[19] Succinctly, the apology symbolized the nation's first official step in acknowledging a) the legal and moral wrongness of the Study, b) the survivors' testimonies,[20] and c) the Tuskegee Legacy Committee's Presidential Apology request.[19] The Study and Clinton's apology for it point to white America's often taken-for-granted malevolent (i.e., subverted beneficent) practices of racism, classism, and sexism in medical science. Clinton's apology certainly accented the unjust racial ethos that fostered racist medicine.

In racist America, whites have scientifically, under the rubric of paternalism, claimed to know what is best for blacks. This false premise required whites to subjugate and maintain blacks socioeconomically, placating them perennially with benevolent and beneficent gestures. Such benevolent and beneficent conditioning made blacks the more vulnerable to whites' racist methods of medical research.[21] It demanded of blacks extraordinary sacrifice so as to prove themselves worthy in the eyes of whites. Whites' forged linkage of science, race, religion, benevolence and beneficence contributed to the making of America's intractable racist ethos that would make the Tuskegee Syphilis Study possible.

THE QUESTION OF SCIENCE, RACE, RELIGION AND BENEVOLENCE

The idea of pseudoscience, race, benevolence, and beneficence dominated the American culture for the forty-year duration of the Study, particularly in the South. The racially segregated South produced the racist ideological soil that nurtured the prejudices of the researchers who conducted the Study. Also, it produced the vulnerability of its victims. Advocates of pseudoscience, race, and subversive versions of benevolence and beneficence perpetuated the myth of the scientific inferiority of blacks. Currying the favor of segregationists, white scientists created malevolent narratives stereotyping blacks as naturally inferior to whites universally. The primary objective of these subversive racist accounts was to characterize blacks as being by nature less than human, functionally unfit to measure up to "Anglo-Saxon-defined civilized standards."

In lieu of the above belief, Anglo-Saxons could argue for almost a century, from the late 19th and early 20th centuries that emancipation had a negative effect upon the health of blacks. Allen Brandt, Harvard professor, noted in his excellent essay written in 1978 shortly following the public disclaimer of the Study: "Physicians studying the effects of emancipation on health concluded almost universally that freedom has caused the mental, moral, and physical deterioration of the black population."[22] White physicians, from slavery through the period of segregation, posited this argument to justify segregating blacks from whites under the legal canopy of white paternalism. Academics of medicine, in such publications as the *Journal of the American Medical Association*, portrayed blacks as sexual perverts who were unfit for the white man's civilization. As one doctor explained in that journal of medicine: "The negro springs from a Southern climate, and as a result his sexual appetite, all of his environment stimulates this appetite, and as a general rule his emotional type religion certainly does not decrease it"[23] Booker T. Washington fell prey to this interpretation of black folk religion, believing that it was an enemy in his race's progress.[24]

The black man became white America's poster child of both diseases and immorality. Bible-thumping Southern evangelical whites explained black skin as originating from the biblical account of Noah cursing his son following the epic Flood. Fallaciously armed, advocates of this biblical view argued that God equated the blackness of the African's skin with being sin flawed.

For generations white evangelical church leaders colluded with their scientific counterparts, particularly in the South, to create malevolent narratives, justifying blacks' degenerative social status.

The ethos of the South in which the Study took place was formed out of ideas, as noted above, from Southern evangelical Christianity and New England Puritan morality to Northern industrial views of beneficence and benevolence toward blacks. Also, black folk religionists' views of *willing the good* and *doing good* within the parameters of the South's racist social structures contributed to this lived world. Major scholars of the Tuskegee Syphilis Study have given very little critical attention to the different religious and moral layers of the Southern ethos in the decades preceding and during the Study. Of all the writers on the subject, James Jones, in his book *Bad Blood*[25] seemingly remained more sensitive to the layered moral factors of the lived world of the Jim Crow South. Susan Reverby, in her fully documented publications, shows a lesser interest in the religious world of the Study on either side of the race divide, as she focuses on the functional value of the folk religion of the more contemporary group of blacks. Reverby's citing of the functional value of the black rural church takes place as a result of her experience in the Shiloh Baptist Church in Nostasulga, Alabama, where she spoke on an occasion to honor the victims of the Study.[26] While recognizing the power of ritual and memory in the black church, Reverby does not address the spirit of hospitality and the show of benevolence that typifies the gathering of black people in a rural church.

Interviewers of the survivors of the Study in later years gave practically no attention to the moral strength of the men and the black religious folk beliefs that undergirded their lived world, particularly their perspectives on health, sin and healing. Many of the black men of this worldview, when the Study was initiated, embraced a view of love and forgiveness that was practically surreal. Herman Shaw's testimony attests to the religious and moral strength of the people of his lived world, as he was one of the original study cohort in 1932 who survived and not only attended Clinton's Presidential Apology at the White House in 1997 but also, at age 95, was a featured speaker at that event. Responding to an interviewer's query of what the Study has possibly done to his faith in his country, Shaw observed to the interviewer on his ninetieth year:

I don't believe I can ever accept the reality of what has happened. However, through the grace of God I will weather the storm and arrive at the point where my country attempts to apologize for their error. Finally, compensation is not real to me. . . . I do whatever I can be worthy of God and my country. It is good however that someone cared. I do whatever I can for my country. It is good to know that someone cared. Somehow it makes all that did happen a little easier to understand.[27]

Shaw's spirit of benevolence and beneficence toward his country is unbeliev-able despite knowing that he and the other men had been used. Such testi-mony from the victim provokes the question of the good consequences from the Study.

THE QUESTION OF THE GOOD OF THE STUDY

Consequentialism, as its name suggests, is primarily concerned with evalu-ating activities with respect to their results. A study of the horizons of benef-icence as it relates to the Tuskegee Syphilis Study in Macon County would be incomplete without critical ethical reflections. What is the consequential good derivable from this Study? This is a generationally haunting question. It is no less applicable for the Study than it has been of previous historical tragedies—a classic example is Nazi Germany's criminal medical experi-ments on the Jewish people. The interest here is not to engage in the debate questions of the moral nuances of the Study's outcome as the literature of moral philosophy shows debates of the Consequentialism theory can be unending. For that reason, the major ethical concern here is: What has been and still ought to be the proper response to the infamous Study? The major contention here is that white bioethicists' responses to the Study must ex-ceed public formalities of expressed sorrows—a mere acknowledging of it as racist—for that only constitutes benevolence, not beneficence. Acknowl-edging alone the fact that the public disclaimer of the Study initiated the burgeoning of the field of bioethics is not enough from white bioethicists, as that again only demonstrates benevolence. Beyond public statements of benevolence, white bioethicists must broaden and deepen their socio-ethical discourses by undertaking overt acts demonstrating their newfound applications of beneficence, actions that tangibly demonstrate them *doing the good*, as distinguished from merely *willing the good*.

One such act of beneficence, on an immediate agenda item, would be for white bioethicists—as a collective voice—to partner with Tuskegee Univer-sity to strengthen its National Center for Bioethics Research in Health Care, as established over a decade ago by President Clinton in his White House Apology. Scholars of beneficent philosophy ought to partner with Tuskegee University to attract private and public funds to preserve this special Bioeth-ics Center place intentionally at the site of the Study. Failure on the part of white bioethicists to do this provokes the painful question: Has Tuskegee, as it relates to the Study at this point in history, become merely a metaphor of academic usury in white bioethical discourse? If so, white bioethicists will merely view Tuskegee's Bioethics Center as a mere benevolent stepchild of the federal government. Well wishes from very influential white bioethicists are inadequate in the face of the Center's continual funding challenges. Rather, white bioethicists' social and professional influence with private and public donors ought to leverage support to maintain this unique National Center for Bioethics Research in Health Care, placed originally so purposefully at the historical epicenter of its founding event.

Allowing this unique Bioethics Center, among the Bioethics Centers that have subsequently been spawned around the country at major universities, to die a slow death for the lack of strong financial support might be viewed as another expression of American racism and classism. Currently, academics in bioethics routinely reference the Tuskegee Study when the issue of "informed consent" is broached. They are no less reluctant in citing the 1974 National Research Act, which mandated the establishment of local institutional review boards for all federally funded research, another legacy from the Tuskegee Syphilis Study. All of these federal regulations are seen as positive derivations of a national constructive response to the tragic Tuskegee Syphilis Study. Susan Reverby has brilliantly summarized different mentionings of the Study in bioethical literature and the value they have for the academic community.[16,17] In short, the Study has become the source of narratives and counternarratives in the culture in general. Charles Rosenberg credits the Study's entry into the American lore as fueling the growth of the "bioethics enterprise."[28]

CONCLUSION

This essay has sought to show that rethinking beneficence and benevolence, from a socio-ethical perspective, is necessary for healthy bioethical discourse. An attempt here has been to demonstrate the thesis by making the United States Public Health Service's infamous Syphilis Study at Tuskegee, starting in 1932 and lasting until 1972, the illustrative fact. Minimally, the following three ethical questions are at the heart of the Study: a) The question of President Clinton's apology; b) The question of pseudoscience, race, religion, and beneficence; and c) the question of consequential good from the Study. Thus the Tuskegee Syphilis Study should prolong the discourse around the ethical challenge of *doing bad* leading to *good results.* It will further show that Tuskegee, where the syphilis study took place, must become more than a metaphor for intellectual usury by bioethicists. The greater future challenge is to make the National Center for Bioethics Research in Health Care at Tuskegee University not only an intellectual place for doing scholarly good but also more richly a means for expanding the horizons of beneficence in public discourse and an overt act itself of beneficence among the nation's bioethicists.

Riggins R. Earl Jr., BA, MDiv, PhD (professor of ethics and theology, Interdenominational Theological Center Atlanta), is an ethicist who has focused his research, writing and teaching on the ethical life of blacks in America. Earl seeks to show how the experiences of racism, classism and genderism, as expressed through slavery and segregation, framed the context for blacks' ethical responses; his book on this theme is Dark Symbols, Obscure Signs: God, Self, and Community in the Slave Mind. *Having published an article on the ethics of the Tuskegee Syphilis Study, he is now writing a book on that topic.*

NOTES

1. Robert Veatch, *The Basics of Bioethics.* 2nd edition. Upper Saddle River, NJ: Prentice Hall, 2003, p. 6–7. For an African American theoretical perspective of values see Peter Paris, *Virtue and Values: The African American Experience.* Minneapolis: Augusburg Fortress, 2004.

2. My theoretical understanding of the phrase "narrative voice" has been influenced greatly by the philosopher Paul Ricouer. See Ricouer's work on narrative ethics. I am interested in the ethics of the narrative. I noted in bioethical literature that the interest in narrative is confined to the clinical setting.

3. Karen LaBacqz "Bio-ethics: Some Challenges from a Liberation Perspective," in *On Moral Medicine: Theological Perspectives in Medical Ethics.* Stephen E. Lammers and Allen Verhey, eds. Grand Rapids, Michigan: Wm. B. Erdmans Publishing Co., 1987, 83.

4. Edmund D. Pellegrino and David C. Thomasma. *For the Patient's Good: The Restoration of Beneficence Health Care.* New York: Oxford University Press, 1988.

5. While the bioethics literature is lacking on the narrative voices of race, class, and gender, this is not the case in social ethics. Emilie Townes's book *Breaking The Fine Rain of Death: African American Health Issues and a Womanist Ethic of Care.* Eugene, Oregon: Wipf & Stock Publishers, 2006. (Previously published by Continuum Publishers, 1998.)

6. For an excellent scholarly account of the evolutionary development of bioethics (before bioethics, the birth of bioethics, after bioethics and beyond bioethics), see Joel James Shuman's *The Body of Compassion: Ethics, Medicine and the Church.* Boulder, Colorado, 1999.

7. Gibson Winter. *Elements for a Social Ethic: Scientific and Ethical Perspectives on Social Process.* New York: Macmillan, 1966.

8. Samuel K. Roberts. In addition to Emilie Townes mentioned below, see the syphilis study in his book *African American Christian Ethics.* Cleveland: Pilgrim Press, 2001.

9. Catherine Myser. "Differences from Somewhere: The Normativity of Whiteness in Bioethics in the United States." *American Journal of Bioethics.* See also Annette Dula. "Whitewashing Black Health: Lies, Deceptions, Assumptions, and Assertions—and the Disparities Continue." In *African American Bioethics: Culture, Race and Identity,* editors Lawrence Prograis Jr. and Edmund D. Pellegrino. Washington, D.C: Georgetown University Press, 2007.

10. United States Public Health Service was the federal agency that conducted the syphilis study at the John Andrews Hospital on the campus of what was then Tuskegee Institute (it later became Tuskegee University) from 1932 to 1972. Practically all scholarly publications merely refer to the infamous study as The Tuskegee Syphilis Study, which is offensive to the members of the Tuskegee University family. It is for this reason I suggest that leaders of the Bioethics Center need to commission a group of scholars to do scholarly study resulting in a signal publication on *the phenomenon of a name*. In other words, the Center must become a dominant voice in the public discourses of the Study. The Center must hold a national forum on this issue.

11. Op. cit., Townes, p. 81–106.

12. Joseph A. Conforti. *Jonathan Edwards, Religious Tradition, and American Culture*. Chapel Hill: University of North Carolina Press, 1995.

13. Eugene Genovese. *Roll, Jordan, Roll: The World the Slaves Made*. New York.

14. Samuel Hopkins. *A Dialogue concerning the Slavery of the Africans, showing it to be the Duty and Interest of American States to emancipate all their African Slaves* (1776). Charles R. Biggs, "Samuel Hopkins and Slavery": http:/www.aplacefortruth .org/Hopkins.htm.

15. See Winthrop D. Jordan. *White Over Black: American Attitudes Toward the Negro, 1550–1812*. Chapel Hill: The University of North Carolina Press, 1995.

16. This apology is cited in Susan Reverby's *Tuskegee's Truth: Rethinking the Tuskegee Syphilis Study*, Chapel Hill: The University of North Carolina Press, 2000, 574–577. This prize-winning book also contains collections of scholarly articles, from an array of scholars, on the Tuskegee Study.

17. Susan M. Reverby, *Examining Tuskegee: The Infamous Syphilis Study and Its Legacy*. Chapel Hill: The University of North Carolina Press, 2009: 225.

18. James Jones, *Bad Blood: The Tuskegee Syphilis Experiment*. New York: Free Press, 1981, Revised Edition, 1992. Jones was the first writer to place the Tuskegee Study in the historical context of American racism. Trained as a historian of medicine, Jones showed how white racism and paternalism produced the ethos for the tragic making of the syphilis study.

19. The Tuskegee Legacy Committee was appointed in 1996. For the chairs and names of the committee, see *Tuskegee's Truth: Rethinking the Tuskegee Syphilis Study*. Edited by Susan Reverby. 559–566.

20. Several manuscripts of the survivors' testimonies were preserved for which we are grateful. Unfortunately, there are serious questions about the questions used to interview the survivors. One of the main concerns is that the framers of the questions seemingly had very little appreciation for the complex worldview of the victims of the study.

21. Previous scholarly studies of the Tuskegee tragedy have not placed it in the historical context of the literature on benevolence, race, class, and gender. Scholars of this literature have contributed greatly to our understanding of the practice of benevolence during the Progressive era. Careful review of the primary and secondary sources on Northern white philanthropy illuminates the role that philanthropists played in shaping the moral dimension of race relations in America. One of the most illuminating secondary sources on the Tuskegee Institute and Northern white

philanthropy was Henry S. Enck's "Tuskegee and Northern White Philanthropy: A Case Study in Fund Raising, 1900–1915." In *The Journal of Negro History*, 65(4) (Autumn, 1980), 336–346.

22. Allan M. Brandt. "Racism and Research: The Case of the Tuskegee Syphilis Experiment." In *Tuskegee's Truths: Rethinking the Tuskegee Syphilis Study*. Edited by Susan M. Reverby, Chapel Hill: The University of North Carolina Press, 2000: 17.

23. H. H. Hazen "Syphilis in the American Negro." In *JAMA*, Aug. 8, 1914: 463.

24. Booker T. Washington, "The Colored Ministry: Its Deficits and Needs," *Christian Union*, 42 (August 14, 1890): 199–200; Louis R. Harlan et al., *The Booker T. Washington Papers* (14 vols.): Urbana, 1972–1989, III.

25. Jones, op. cit.

26. Reverby, op. cit., 239.

27. Deadly Deception Complete Interviews, Schlesinger Library Radcliffe College, Cambridge, Massachusetts, unpublished, 1977, Nova—Tuskegee SR 19, pages 41–42, Herman Shaw Interview.

28. Charles E. Rosenberg. "Meanings, Policies and Medicine: On the Bioethical Enterprise and History." *Daedalus 128* (Fall 1999): 27–46.

Essay 13

Medicine, Research, and Socio-Cultural History

Reciprocal Relationships

Virginia M. Brennan

Health and illness are complex phenomena, involving not only organic conditions but the socio-cultural context in which people live. What counts as health or illness in one society does not in another: for example, Akyeampong notes that in Ghana, a woman who is barren is traditionally seen as being ill, but this is not the 21st-century Western medical view.[1]

Furthermore, historical events can exert an influence on how people understand and feel about current events, including medical care and biomedical research, and thus have a bearing on their well-being. Perhaps the most famous example of such a relationship today is between the 40-year Tuskegee Syphilis Study and the willingness of African Americans to participate in biomedical research: In this case, the unethical research program to which African American men with syphilis were subjected between 1930 and 1970 appears to have left in its wake distrust of biomedical research in the African American community today.[2–15]

Conversely, the socio-cultural context in which research is conducted and medicine practiced has a bearing on their results. In approaches to the history of medicine that make this their starting point, the biomedical formulation of health and illness themselves are scrutinized in terms of the social structures and culture in which that formulation took place. A leading medical historian who helped develop the so-called new social history of medicine is Charles E. Rosenberg, who has written about such phenomena as 19th-century understandings of cholera;[16] the mental health of Charles Julius Guiteau, the man who assassinated James Garfield;[17] and the rise of hospitals,[18] all in the

United States. Social history of medicine frames health, illness, and medicine in terms of gender, race, ethnicity, and class. As Reverby and Rosner put it, social history of medicine goes "beyond the great doctors" to look critically at the formulation of health and illness in terms of the dominant paradigms of everyday life in the period being studied, thus objectifying them as historical phenomena, to be understood in the same terms in which art, politics, and domestic life can be understood.[19,20]

The history of medicine evolved further with the cultural turn of the postmodern era. Cultural history of medicine is informed by "anthropology, cultural materialism, the history of *mentalités,* and so forth" and blossomed in the late 1970s and 1980s[21] (p. 365). Cultural historians took from the seminal work of anthropologist Clifford Geertz[22] "the idea that an event could be read like a text, that a riot or a parade or a massacre of cats or other nonliterary production had symbolic meanings that a historian could recover and analyze"[21] (p. 368). Rosenberg was influential in the development of the cultural history of medicine as well.[23]

A good recent example of social history comes from the work of sociologist Elizabeth M. Armstrong,[25–27] who has written extensively about fetal alcohol syndrome, first identified (and named) in 1973 by Jones and Smith.[28]

PART I: HISTORY AND TRUST

Before turning to social history of medicine in the U.S., I would like to make one point about the converse relationship between historical events and contemporary attitudes and beliefs: My one point is that the relationship between historical facts and contemporary beliefs and attitudes can be strong and long-lasting, even when it is indirect. One is more likely to have accurate knowledge of events that one witnesses, or that one hears of from contemporaries who were witnesses, than one is to have of events whose details have been passed down across generations. Such accurate knowledge, however, is not necessary for the imparted memory of the events to influence people's attitudes and beliefs. This example (from outside the realm of medicine) demonstrates how very long-lasting such indirect effects can be: according a recent analysis by a team of economists, there are elevated rates of distrust in African ethnolinguistic communities whose ancestors were disproportionately victimized by the slave trade centuries ago.[29]

In the realm of medicine, a RAND study[30] reports that a large proportion of African American respondents endorsed one or more forms of a conspiracy theory regarding AIDS and its effects on black America; in light of the long history of ill treatment of African Americans at the hands of both biomedical researchers and health professionals, skepticism about the source of a virulent disease having disproportionate effects on the black community seems unsurprising[2-16] (pp. 31–36).

General distrust of biomedical researchers and health professionals might characterize a culture as a result of a long history of harm without detailed knowledge of the historical events being widespread in the culture. Conflicting accounts of levels of trust in biomedical researchers and willingness to participate in biomedical research[2-16] (pp. 31–36) may be due to differences in the research with respect to whether or not specific historical knowledge was a criterion.

Two additional examples underscore the fact that the relationship between historical facts and contemporary beliefs and attitudes is strong and long-lasting, even when it is indirect. One concerns the death of the renowned black physician Charles R. Drew at a hospital in the South in 1950, and the other concerns the catastrophic flooding of New Orleans in the aftermath of Hurricane Katrina in 2005.

Dr. Charles R. Drew, an African American physician and researcher, was instrumental in the development of blood banks on a large scale during World War II, which enabled medical staff to save many lives during the war. A professor at Howard University Medical School, Drew died in a car crash in rural Alamance County, North Carolina in 1950 while traveling with colleagues to Tuskegee, Alabama, for an annual free clinic. While Drew was not killed immediately in the crash, he died in a nearby hospital despite intense medical efforts to save him, according to one of his colleagues who survived the crash.[37] Subsequently the story that Drew had died because treatment was withheld from him due to his race became widespread. Love (1997) writes,

> Within hours, a rumor about the accident began to travel: Drew had bled to death because a local hospital had refused to treat him because he was black. Over a period of years, the story became a full-fledged historical legend, dramatizing the bitter irony embedded in black history. In 1964, at the height of the civil rights movement, Whitney Young wrote a column about segregated medical care that employed the Drew legend as a dramatic example of mistreatment. Soon the legend was printed in other newspapers, in magazines, and in history books. It was featured on television shows: the man who had "discovered" blood plasma and had saved countless lives by setting up the World War II blood collection program had been refused blood. The story is still widely believed today [pp. 1–2].[37]

Why did the story of Drew's tragic death transform itself into this particular legendary form? The history of racialized medical care in the U.S., and in particular the history of hospitals, goes a long way toward an explanation. As studied most extensively in Gamble's 1995 book, *Making a Place for Ourselves: The Black Hospital Movement, 1920–1945*,[33] and also in Byrd and Clayton's monumental history of race and medicine in the U.S.,[31] hospital care was rigidly denied to people of color, or provided only in hospitals or inferior wards set apart for people of color, from the time that U.S. hospitals were first founded (in the 18th century) well into the 20th century. Such racialized medicine was in full swing during Dr. Drew's career. To use just one example, we note that Drew was a stalwart campaigner against the practice of segregating stored blood on the basis of the race of the donor, which was widespread in the mid-20th century.

Drawing the connection between this racialized historical context and the legend that arose upon Dr. Drew's death, Love continues,

> As this study demonstrates, there are different kinds of historical truth, and the history that people pass on orally—a group's legends—is an important clue not only to how they feel and think about their past but also to the very substance of that past. . . . The Drew legend is not literally true, but it reveals a large truth at the heart of black culture: it demonstrates the continuing psychological trauma of segregation and racism in American life. . . . The legend's message is that even if you are Charles Drew, a great man by any standard, you will not be treated appropriately in twentieth-century America. The legend speaks for the many undocumented experiences of black Americans whose medical treatment was delayed or denied because of white racism [pp. 4–6][37]

Another example of the powerful connections between history and contemporary beliefs and attitudes concerns the broken levees that flooded the heavily African American Ninth Ward of New Orleans after Hurricane Katrina in late August and early September of 2005. Cordasco and colleagues[38] report on a belief among survivors of the flood in New Orleans that authorities had deliberately blown up the levee bordering the Ninth Ward that held back the massive waters that embrace the city. As Cordasco and colleagues note, such a belief was likely rooted in historical rather than contemporary fact.

In the great Mississippi River flood of 1927, New Orleans's leaders did in fact deliberately dynamite a levee and flood. On April 29th, the flood having reached the vicinity of New Orleans, the city spent $2 million to dynamite the Poydras levee, blasting a break of 1,500 feet that sent the water cascading away from town. The flood ran as the lead story in the nation's newspapers for weeks. Although the risk to New Orleans from the flood that had devastated the Midwest and Upper South was by that point small, the city fathers chose to flood much of St. Bernard Parish and all of Plaquemines Parish's east bank as a means of reassuring investors that the City of New Orleans remained as viable as ever. Although those leaders promised the residents of the flooded parishes that they would reimburse them for the losses of their homes and livelihoods, in fact they fought hard in court not to do so, and in the end never did.[39]

This travesty in the treatment of the people at the hands of the authorities appears to have left its mark on the minds of low-income people in New Orleans. Ultimately, more than 1,800 people died as a result of the storm and subsequent flooding, many because they failed to evacuate despite warnings from authorities to do so.[40] Cordasco and colleagues interviewed more than 50 survivors of Hurricane Katrina in New Orleans and argue that distrust underlay the decision of many low-income New Orleans residents not to evacuate. They report:

> A striking element of distrust expressed by interviewees was perceived dishonesty, or a lack of truthfulness and sincerity. Eight people we interviewed did not believe the reports in the media and claims of the authorities that the flooding in their neighborhoods came from the levees being overwhelmed by storm waters. Two people stated that they believed that the water was diverted into the poor neighborhoods to save the rich neighborhoods. Explaining how "the politicians broke the pump," one individual said: "They let the waters go in the poor neighborhoods and kept it out of the rich neighborhoods, like that French Quarter where tourists go at." Six people went further and stated that they believed that the levees were intentionally broken. One person stated, "He sacrificed New Orleans. He cut that 17th bridge, because you've got to sacrifice something. Donald Trump is putting the tower on Canal Street downtown and they saved the French Quarter and the Garden District, the historical areas, the rich people, where the money is coming from, casinos and all that. And they drowned out all the poor people and the lower-middle class working people . . . And they do that all over the country, not just in New Orleans . . . they do stuff and then they lie, lie, lie" [p. 279: journal pagination].[38]

In all of these instances, historically real harm (the slave trade,[28] nontherapeutic experimentation on human beings,[4,34,36] unauthorized autopsies on cadavers of African Americans,[32–36] the Tuskegee Syphilis Study,[2–15] the segregation of hospitals,[31,33] and the dynamiting of the New Orleans levee in 1927[39]) has yielded practical consequences for the descendents of those harmed. These earlier events live on in present-day distrust, unwillingness to participate in biomedical research, discomfort with the health care system and practitioners, and people's disregard of warnings issued by government authorities, among other things.

PART II: MEDICINE AS A SOCIO-CULTURAL ARTIFACT

The influence of historical events on the delivery of medical care and public health in the present day is matched by influence running in the opposite direction: the socio-cultural context in which medicine is practiced and medical science takes shape influences both how health and illness are understood and how they are treated. This is addressed in the second part of this essay.

Social and cultural history open up to critical analysis not only the practice and delivery of health care, but medical knowledge itself.[21,26,41,42] Brandt expressed the central notion of this paradigm as it relates to the identification of diseases as follows:

> Fundamental to the notion that disease is socially constructed is the premise that it is profoundly shaped by both biological and cultural variables. Attitudes and values concerning disease affect the perception of its pattern of transmission, its epidemiological nature. Only if we understand the way disease is influenced by social and cultural forces—issues of class, race, ethnicity, and gender—can we effectively address its biological dimension. A "social construction" reveals tacit values, it becomes a symbol for ordering and explaining aspects of the human experience. In this light, medicine is not just affected by social, economic, and political variables—it is embedded in them [p. 5].[41]

In what follows, I will comment on the evolving social construction of mental illness and alcoholism in the United States.

Since the founding of the U.S., immigrant groups have often been associated in both the popular press and the professional literature as being the source of specific infectious diseases and as being disproportionately characterized by such conditions as mental illness, addiction, and alcoholism.[18,41,43-45] Kraut writes,

> The menace of diseases from afar, borne by the bodies of immigrants and refugees, and the American public's response to that possibility have been intertwined with nativism and ethnic prejudice throughout American history. . . . Always, Americans have believed immigrants posed a threat. They have feared that poor health and frail physiques might make of immigrants burdens rather than assets; might spread infectious diseases among the native-born, undermining the advantages of the very society that offered freedom and opportunity to those who could find it nowhere else.

> Historians of immigration and historians of medicine have only begun to explore the linkages between nativism and the social construction of health and disease in different eras of American history. One such study treating the mid-nineteenth century is Charles Rosenberg's now-classic volume, *The Cholera Years*. Rosenberg demonstrates how nativists in New York City stigmatized Irish immigrants with responsibility for this dreaded infectious disease, a disease that was actually triggered by living conditions in the host nation. In Rosenberg's study the voice of nativist prejudice is unmistakable. Similarly, historian of medicine Gerald Grob has described how mental illness of institutionalized Irish immigrants was attributed to an inherent instability characteristic of the

new arrivals. In both instances, disease was socially constructed by nativists to stigmatize Irish immigrants [p. 154].[44]

Tracy, who also discusses the widespread association of inebriation and mental illness with immigrant groups in the United States in the late 19th and early 20th centuries, argues that physicians' self-interest played a role in establishing the view of alcoholism as a disease.[46] In the late 19th century, specialization began to increase the value of physicians' services; as part of this trend, specialties in public health and psychiatry—both of which dealt extensively with people impaired by excessive use of alcohol—emerged in the early 20th century. While mental illnesses and limitations that were not associated with substance use often proved intractable, physicians had more hope of success when they could straightforwardly remove the proximal cause of the illness (i.e., alcohol). (See also Lunbeck on the development of psychiatry in the U.S. in the Progressive Era.[47])

In a helpful discussion of the shifting terminology for what is today called alcoholism, Tracy notes that the term dipsomania tended to be attached to excessive drinkers of the middle and upper classes.[46] That is, the term (which implied that the condition was psychiatric, analogous to kleptomania and monomania) was applied differentially based on social class. The psychiatric connotations of the term dipsomania contrasted with the moral censure implicit in the terms intemperance and habitual drunkenness. Crowley and White discuss the uneven application of the disease model of alcoholism in the 19th century this way:

> It should be noted, however, that this new definition of the inebriate as someone worthy of rescue had its limitations. First, the medical model of inebriety was extended primarily to men, not to women, whose excessive alcohol consumption continued throughout the nineteenth century to be defined almost exclusively in moral terms. There were also class distinctions. The set of those worthy to be rescued was restricted primarily to men of means who, after achieving some degree of success in life, had fallen on hard times as a direct consequence of alcoholism. Those of less wealth and less noble histories were more likely to be viewed not as inebriates worthy of rescue but as "common sots" [p. 8].[48]

As suggested here, the pathology of alcoholism was deemed to coincide not only with immigrant status/ethnic group membership and social class, but also with gender. In the late 19th and early 20th century, the common view was that habitual drunkenness was less common among women than among men, but somehow worse when it did occur. Tracy quotes the municipal physicians of Boston in 1919 as saying that addiction to alcohol in women "means a further step downward than it does with men. . . . [W]e should expect to find among women taken up from the streets and from cafes because of drunkenness a larger percentage of mental defect and disorder."[49]

The temperance movement in the U.S. has historically been a feminine enterprise,[47] a fact that was very much in keeping with the popular perception of the intemperate drinker as a particular masculine type: a brutal man, given to neglecting his children and beating up his wife. As Lunbeck writes of how the word was used in the Progressive Era, "'Drunkard' was no mere description but, rather, a heavily freighted image forged in the heat of public, politicized sexual antagonism."[47] (p. 244)

From all directions, then, society in the late 19th and early 20th century stigmatized habitual drunkenness. At the same time, reformers (many of them physicians) recast it from being a moral failing to being a disease, subject to medical intervention and therapy. Even in its new incarnation as a disease, however, corrosive characteristics attached themselves to the concept of the disorder: the superintendant of St. Elizabeth's Hospital for the Insane, W. W. Godding, opined in 1887 that society required protection "against that race deterioration—those inherited neuroses, chorea, epilepsy, idiocy and insanity—of offspring begotten in a debauch" (quoted p. 59, Tracy, 2005).[50] In the early 20th century, physicians and medical societies recommended that alcoholics be prevented from procreating, and they were subject to incarceration in workhouses, asylums, and jails. (Also see Lunbeck on eugenics in relation to psychiatry in the first decades of the 20th century.[47])

CONCLUSION

In this essay we have taken a bird's-eye view in order to observe the reciprocity of the relationships among medicine, research, and socio-cultural history. First, we saw how the past inexorably exerts its influence on present-day knowledge, attitudes, and behavior, even when the inherited knowledge of past events has been altered as the stories are told and retold over generations. We saw that historical events—the slave trade,[29] nontherapeutic experimentation on human beings,[4,34,36] unauthorized autopsies on cadavers of African Americans,[32-36] the Tuskegee Syphilis Study,[2-15] the segregation of hospitals,[31,33] and the dynamiting of the New Orleans levee in 1927[39]—live on in the collective memory of descendents of those harmed. In the second part of this essay, we looked at the reciprocal relationship: socio-cultural context influences how particular medical conditions are understood and treated. In all of these instances, we are reminded to approach the business of understanding public health with a respectful awareness of the richness and complexity of all peoples' collective and personal identity.

Virginia Brennan, PhD, MA, has been the editor of the Journal of Health Care for the Poor and Underserved *since 2001. She is a member of the faculty of Meharry Medical College. She is the editor of and a contributor to the book* Natural Disasters and Public Health: Hurricanes Katrina, Rita, and Wilma *(Johns Hopkins University Press, 2009) and of another book (on free clinics) scheduled for publication in Winter 2011/2012. She was previously a faculty member in linguistics and psychology at Swarthmore College and Vanderbilt University.*

NOTES

1. Akyeampong, E. Alcoholism in Ghana—A sociocultural exploration. *Culture, Medicine, and Psychiatry* 1995, 19:261–280.

2. Gamble, V. N. Under the shadow of Tuskegee: African Americans and health care. *AJPH* 1997 Nov., 87(11): 1773–1778.

3. Jacobs, E. A., Rolle, I., Ferrans, C. E., Whitaker, E. E., and Warnecke, R. B. Understanding African Americans' views of the trustworthiness of physicians. *J Gen Intern Med.* 2006 Jun., 21(6):642–7.

4. Lederer, S. E. The Tuskegee syphilis experiment and the conventions and practice of biomedical research. In Warner, J. H., and Tighe, J. A., eds. *Major Problems in the History of American Medicine and Public Health: Documents and Essays.* Boston and New York: Houghton Mifflin Company, 2001.

5. Reverby, S. M., ed. *Tuskegee's Truths: Rethinking the Tuskegee Syphilis Study.* Chapel Hill, NC: University of North Carolina Press, 2000.

6. Sade, R. M.. Publication of unethical research studies: The importance of informed consent. *Ann Thorac Surg.* 2003 Feb., 75(2):325–8.

7. Shavers, V. L., Lynch, C. F., and Burmeister, L. F. Knowledge of the Tuskegee Study and its impact on the willingness to participate in medical research studies. *JNMA* 2000 Dec., 92(12): 563–572.

8. Shavers, V. L., Lynch, C. F., and Burmeister, L. F. Racial differences in factors that influence the willingness to participate in medical research studies. *Ann Epidemiol* 2002 May, 12(4):248–256.

9. Wendler, D., Kington, R., Madans, S., et al. Are racial and ethnic minorities less willing to participate in health research? *PLoS Medicine,* 2006 Feb., 3(2)201–210.

10. Wynia, M. K., and Gamble, V. N. Mistrust among minorities and the trustworthiness of medicine, letter in response to Wendler et al. *PLoS Medicine,* 2006 May, 3(5): 701–2.

11. Katz, R. V., Green, B. L., Kressin, N. R., et al. The legacy of the Tuskegee syphilis study: Assessing its impact on willingness to participate in biomedical studies. *J Health Care Poor Underserved* 19.4 2008 Nov., 1169–81.

12. Katz, R. V., Kegeles, S. S., Kressin, N. R., et al. The Tuskegee Legacy Project: Willingness of minorities to participate in biomedical research. *J Health Care Poor Underserved* 2006 Nov., 17(4):698–715.

13. McCallum, J. M., Arekere, D. M., Green, B. L., et al. Awareness and knowledge of the U.S. Public Health Service Syphilis Study at Tuskegee: Implications for biomedical research. *J Health Care Poor Underserved* Nov. 2006, 17(4):716–733.

14. Scharff, D., Mathews, K. J., Williams, M., et al. More than Tuskegee: Understanding mistrust about research participation. *J Health Care Poor Underserved* Aug. 2010, 21(3): 879–97.

15. Carter, V. L., and Coby, N. *Journal of Health Care for the Poor and Underserved* (*JHCPU*) supplemental issue sponsored by the Tuskegee University National Center for Bioethics in Research and Health Care and the Historically Black Colleges and Universities Research Network. *JHCPU* Aug. 2010, 21(3 Suppl).

16. Rosenberg, C. E. *The Cholera Years: The United States in 1832, 1849, and 1866.* Chicago: The University of Chicago Press, 1962.

17. Rosenberg, C. E. *The Trial of the Assassin Guiteau: Psychiatry and the Law in the Gilded Age.* Chicago and London: The University of Chicago Press, 1968.

18. Rosenberg, C. E. *The Care of Strangers: The Rise of America's Hospital System.* Basic Books. 1987.

19. Reverby, S., and Rosner, D. Medical culture and historical practice. In Warner, J. H., and Tighe, J. A., eds. *Major Problems in the History of American Medicine and Public Health: Documents and Essays.* Boston and New York: Houghton Mifflin Company, 2001.

20. Reverby, S., and Rosner, D. "Beyond the Great Doctors" revisited: A generation of the "new" social history of medicine. In Huisman, F., and Warner, J. H., eds. *Locating Medical History: The Stories and Their Meanings.* Baltimore: Johns Hopkins University Press, 2004.

21. Fissell, M.. "Making meaning from the margins: The new cultural history of medicine." In Warner, J., and Huisman, F., eds. *Locating Medical History: The Stories and their Meanings.* Baltimore: Johns Hopkins University Press, 2004: 365.

22. Geertz, C. *The Interpretation of Cultures.* New York: Basic Books, 1973.

23. Rosenberg, C. E., and Golden, J., eds. *Framing Disease: Studies in Cultural History.* New Brunswick, N.J.: Rutgers University Press, 1992.

24. Rosenberg is hardly one to dismiss the centrality of biological fact for any history of disease. He writes, for example, "The emergence of AIDS and the intractability of certain psychiatric conditions made visible by the deinstitutionalization movement have both played an important role in underlining the need to factor in biopathological mechanisms in understanding the particular social negotiations that frame particular diseases. Physicians and social scientists concerned with such issues necessarily inhabit what might be called a postrelativist moment; neither biological reductionism nor an exclusive social constructionism constitute viable intellectual positions. Refer to note 23, p. xxiv.

25. Armstrong, E. M. Diagnosing moral disorder: The discovery and evolution of fetal alcohol syndrome. *Soc Sci Med* Dec. 1998, 47(12):2025–42.

26. Armstrong, E. *Conceiving Risk, Bearing Responsibility: Fetal Alcohol Syndrome and the Diagnosis of a Moral Disorder.* Baltimore: Johns Hopkins University Press, 2003.

27. Armstrong, E. M., and Abel, E. L. Fetal alcohol syndrome: the origins of a moral panic. *Alcohol Alcohol.* May–Jun. 2000, 35(3):276–82.

28. Jones, K. L., and Smith, D. W. Recognition of the fetal alcohol syndrome in early infancy. *Lancet.* Nov. 1973, 302(7836):999–1001.

29. Nunn, N., and Wantchekon, L. The slave trade and the origins of mistrust in Africa. The National Bureau of Economics Research (NBER) Working Paper No. 14783, 2009 Mar.

30. Bogart, L. M., and Thorburn, S. Are HIV/AIDS conspiracy beliefs a barrier to HIV prevention among African Americans? *J Acquir Immune Defic Syndr.* Feb. 2005, 1, 38(2):213–18.

31. Byrd, W. M., and Clayton, L. A. *An American Health Dilemma: Race, Medicine, and Health Care in the United States,* Vol. 1: Beginnings to 1900; Vol. 2: 1900–2000. New York and London: Routledge, 2002.

32. Fry, G. M. *Night Riders in Black Folk History.* Athens, Georgia: U. of Georgia Press, 1975 (reprinted as a Brown Thrasher Book in 1991).

33. Gamble, V. N. *Making a Place for Ourselves: The Black Hospital Movement, 1920–1945.* New York: Oxford University Press, 1995.

34. Lederer, S. *Subjected to Science: Human Experimentation in America before the Second World War.* Baltimore: Johns Hopkins University Press, 1995.

35. Rothamn, D. J. The doctor as stranger: Medicine and public distrust. In Warner, J. H., and Tighe, J. A., eds. *Major Problems in the History of American Medicine and Public Health: Documents and Essays.* Boston and New York: Houghton Mifflin Company, 2001.

36. Savitt, T. L. Race, human experimentation, and dissection in the antebellum South. In Warner, J. H., and Tighe, J. A., eds. *Major Problems in the History of American Medicine and Public Health: Documents and Essays.* Boston and New York: Houghton Mifflin Company, 2001.

37. Love, S. *One Blood: The Death and Resurrection of Charles R. Drew.* Chapel Hill: UNC Press, 1997.

38. Cordasco, K. M., Eisenman, D. P., Glik, D. C., et al. "They blew the levee": Distrust of authorities among Hurricane Katrina evacuees. In Brennan, V., ed. *Disasters and Public Health: Hurricanes Katrina, Rita, and Wilma.* Baltimore: Johns Hopkins University Press, 2009.

39. Barry, J. M. *Rising Tide: The Great Mississippi Flood of 1927 and How It Changed America.* New York: Simon & Schuster, 1998.

40. Brennan, V. Introduction. In Brennan, V., ed. *Disasters and Public Health: Hurricanes Katrina, Rita, and Wilma.* Baltimore: Johns Hopkins University Press, 2009.

41. Brandt, A. M. *No Magic Bullet: A Social History of Venereal Disease in the United States Since 1880.* New York, Oxford: Oxford University Press, 1985.

42. Jordanova, L. The social construction of medical knowledge. In Huisman, F., and Warner, J. H., eds. *Locating Medical History: The Stories and Their Meanings.* Baltimore: Johns Hopkins University Press, 2004.

43. Kraut, A. M. Physicians and the new immigration during the Progressive Era. In Warner, J. H., and Tighe, J. A., eds. *Major Problems in the History of American*

Medicine and Public Health: Documents and Essays. Boston and New York: Houghton Mifflin Company, 2001.

44. Kraut, A. M. Illness and medical care among Irish immigrants in antebellum New York. In Bayor, R. H., and Meagher, T. J., eds. *The New York Irish.* Baltimore: Johns Hopkins University Press, 1996.

45. Risse, G. B. Bubonic plague, bacteriology, and anti-Asian racism in San Francisco, 1900. In Warner, J. H., and Tighe, J. A., eds. *Major Problems in the History of American Medicine and Public Health: Documents and Essays.* Boston and New York: Houghton Mifflin Company, 2001.

46. Tracy, S. W. *Alcoholism in America: From Reconstruction to Prohibition.* Baltimore: Johns Hopkins University Press, 2005.

47. Lunbeck, E. *The Psychiatric Persuasion: Knowledge, Gender, and Power in Modern America.* Princeton, NJ: Princeton University Press, 1994.

48. Crowley, J. W., and White, W. L. *Drunkard's Refuge: The Lessons of the New York State Inebriate Asylum.* Amherst: University of Massachusetts Press, 2004.

49. Anderson, V. V., and Leonard, C. M. Drunkenness as seen among women in court. *Mental Hygiene,* 1919, 3:271.

50. W.W. Godding opined in 1887 (Tracy, p. 59).

Essay 14

Healing the Sin-Sick Soul

Reflections on the Syphilis Study

Rueben C. Warren

While the usual response to the U.S. Public Health Service (USPHS) Syphilis Study at Tuskegee generates remorse, guilt, shame, and hopelessness, this essay focuses on hope and healing. Hope, in this context, refers to a high sense of expectation, regardless of history and current circumstances. Healing is a way of releasing power to others rather than holding on to it oneself (Campbell, 1995).[1] This essay reflects the thoughts of one black man, while he was employed at the Centers for Disease Control and Prevention (CDC),[2] about a series of events that preceded his own knowledge—his own acute awareness—of the USPHS Syphilis Study at Tuskegee. Those thoughts, having been initiated by a challenge from an academic colleague in 1994 to encourage a nonresponsive government to apologize for its unethical institutional behavior in conducting the USPHS Syphilis Study at Tuskegee, eventually led to the series of events that swirled into the establishment of the Tuskegee Legacy Committee in 1996. Those same thoughts led to ensuing reflections centered around that black man's heartfelt impressions immediately after the 1997 Presidential Apology and his continuing reflections since the apology on the bioethical and public health ethical issues associated with that sad and tragic study. I am that man.

CONTEXT

The infamous USPHS Syphilis Study at Tuskegee has many titles, descriptions, and other characterizations describing a study about syphilis, a venereal disease, conducted during a time when syphilis was rampant and research scientists were desperately trying to prevent and/or cure it. Some viewed the study as a badly needed public health effort when syphilis was at near epidemic levels in many communities. Others describe it as the most egregious example of misconduct in biomedical research in U.S. history. Still others viewed the USPHS Syphilis Study at Tuskegee as a simple act of institutional racism. The facts vary by storyteller, but what is known is that the study consisted of 399 syphilitic Negro males who never received treatment, 201 nonsyphilitic Negro males, with 275 of these syphilitic Negro males having been given some level of treatment during the first two years of the syphilitic process. Thus the study participants were all black men[3] and their ages ranged between 25 and 39 years when the study began.[4] They all supposedly lived in Macon County, Alabama; some were married and some were not. Their education and income varied even though they were reported as poor and uneducated. Various accounts of the event suggest that that the men knew what was going on and volunteered for various benefits. Others report that the men knew nothing and were intentionally misinformed and misled. While the precise facts may never be fully known, the question is, how reliable and verifiable is what was reported, even published in book after book or in the peer-reviewed scientific literature? Will we ever know the full truth?

In the 1997 Presidential Apology, Bill Clinton apologized to the men and their families and to the African American community. He said, "The United States government did something that was wrong—deeply, profoundly, and morally wrong."[5] Yet, biomedical research and other human health sciences do not traditionally use the language of right or wrong in their vernacular. The language of science uses constructs of valid or invalid, correct or incorrect, statistically significant or insignificant.[6] Consequently, the dilemma in deconstructing the legacy of the USPHS Syphilis Study at Tuskegee transcends biomedical science and research and demands a trans-disciplinary engagement of a diverse group of academicians including clinicians, philosophers, theologians, ethicists, behavioral scientists, public health practitioners and health policy officials. To understand what really happened, those most directly affected by the study must be at the core of the conversations.

The importance of language must be acknowledged when communicating about sensitive past and current events related to the USPHS Syphilis Study at Tuskegee. The men in this study were black. For example, the terms enslaved African, Negro, nonwhite, colored, black, black American, non-Hispanic black, Afro-American, African in America, African American and even the "N" word have been used at various times, for various reasons, to describe the same group of people. Even the Federal Office of Management and Budget (OMB), Directive 15, uses black and African American synonymously when in fact, black refers to race and African American describes an ethnic group among black people.[7] Interestingly even though Egypt is located in North Africa, OMB lists Egyptians as white or Caucasian.[7]

Equally confusing, and confounding all ensuing discussions, is the commonly known and widely used name for this study: "Tuskegee Syphilis Study," which fails to reflect that the U.S. Public Health Service (USPHS), a unit in the U.S. Department of Health and Human Services, officially sponsored the study throughout its entire course of conduct. Even when direct oversight for the study transferred to the CDC in Atlanta, Georgia (then-named as the Communicable Disease Center) in the mid-1960s, the overall responsibility for the study remained with the USPHS until its ending in 1972[4] (p. 75). In 1972, Peter Buxton, a former PHS venereal disease investigator, who had relentlessly raised ethical issues about the Syphilis Study story, discussed his concerns with a reporter in San Francisco. On July 26, 1972, the AP wire release read, "Syphilis Victims in U.S. Went Untreated for 40 Years"[4] (p. 85). Soon afterward, in professional conversations and publications, more importantly in the popular press, the name became "The Tuskegee Syphilis Study."

Vanessa Gamble, MD, PhD, a physician and medical historian and the second Director of the National Center for Bioethics in Research and Health Care at Tuskegee University, while serving as a member of a CDC national advisory council on bioethics, insisted that the name for the study accurately reflect that the primary investigative unit was the U.S. Public Health Service and the federal operating division for oversight was CDC; thus, the title, USPHS Syphilis Study at Tuskegee.[8] Today, on the campus of Tuskegee University and among those most informed and/or engaged in activities related to the study, the term Tuskegee Syphilis Study is not used because it is a misnomer.

The USPHS Syphilis Study at Tuskegee has also been referred to as the Tuskegee Experiment. This title is easily confused with a World War II phenomenon which was entitled the "Tuskegee Experiment." This was an administrative project of the then segregated U.S. military which created a separate unit of black military airplane pilots who, having been trained at what was then Tuskegee Institute, went on to earn military distinction for their service and accomplishments in World War II.

I graduated from the School of Dentistry, Meharry Medical College, in 1972 and for many years, Meharry medical and dental students, residents and some faculty rotated to John A. Andrews Hospital and the Veterans Administration Hospital, both in Tuskegee, Alabama. Having "externed" in urban and rural community health settings throughout dental school and graduate school in public health, I never heard of the "Tuskegee Syphilis Study." In 1988, after joining CDC, as Associate Director for Minority Health (ADMH), I learned about a health insurance program for a group of men in Tuskegee, Alabama, managed by the largest center at CDC, the National Center for Preventive Services. (CPS) The CDC was organized according to either categories of diseases or preventive services provided.[9] The CPS managed research and preventive services for sexually transmitted diseases, tuberculosis, some chronic diseases and support to and for State Health Departments. An African American man, employed at CDC as a Public Health Advisor, managed the insurance program and interacted with the surviving men and their families. We met and he shared all of the background material on the USPHS Syphilis Study at Tuskegee, so I could better understand what led to the insurance program. I also read the book *Bad Blood* by James H. Jones, which was the first major book published on the USPHS Syphilis Study at Tuskegee.[10]

In late 1994, after a telephone call from an academic colleague, Ralph Katz, DMD, MPH PhD, then Director of a National Institute of Dental and Craniofacial Research at the NIH [NIDCR/NIH] Regional Research Center for Minority Oral Health, concerning his belief that this bioethical dilemma called for a public apology, as the ADMH I brought the Syphilis Study issue to the attention of the Director of CDC. The matter was assigned jointly to me as the ADMH and to the Director of CPS, presumably because the men were black and the disease of concern was syphilis.

Early in the 1995–96 federal fiscal year, Clay Simpson, then Director of the DHHS Office of Minority Health and I, as the CDC ADMH, invited a group of people to meet on Tuskegee University's campus to discuss the ethical issues surrounding the USPHS Syphilis Study at Tuskegee. They agreed that a meeting should be held on the campus of Tuskegee University, so those most directly affected could be present. After a series of planning steps, in January 1996 a workshop, jointly funded by the AMDH/CDC and the OMH/DHHS and sponsored by the Minority Health Professions Foundation, convened a trans-disciplinary group of government and nongovernment people at Tuskegee University to discuss what should be done to address this bioethical issue[11] (see details in Katz 2003, as well as in the introduction of this book). The group later named the Tuskegee Legacy Committee was largely formed from the attendees at this workshop and proved instrumental first in developing the concept and details of the eventual Presidential Apology at this workshop, and then in the pushing of it as an agenda item at the national political level.

At that January 1996 workshop, the participants unanimously decided that the federal government should apologize. The essential question was who should apologize on behalf of the "government"? As previously indicated, CDC had assumed oversight over the study in the mid-1960s and they were currently managing the health insurance program for the survivors and their families. It seemed logical that the apology should come from the Director of

CDC. Ironically, the Director of CDC was African American, and an apology from him would appear self-serving and more important, it would not be clear that the matter reached beyond the black population. The injustice was conducted by the U.S federal government and the apology should come from the President. As some of the members of the Tuskegee Legacy Committee were employed at CDC, they could not direct the CDC Director, and surely not the President, to do anything. The Tuskegee Legacy Committee needed persons who would not be jeopardized by their action to provide the leadership for the group. Thus, the committee selected two well-positioned, highly regarded members who were not federal government employees, Drs. Vanessa Gamble and John Fletcher, to co-chair the committee. The request was for the President to apologize for the study and to establish a National Bioethics Center on the campus of Tuskegee University. Among others things, the proposed apology mandated that the focus should be on research, education and service activities to prevent similar occurrences from ever happening again. While the committee felt that the apology should occur on campus in Tuskegee, subsequent political considerations (including the fact that President Clinton was recovering from a surgically repaired knee tendon at the time of the scheduled apology event) led to the final decision to host the apology event at the White House. On May 16, 1997, in the East Room of the White House, Bill Clinton apologized on behalf of the people of the United States and, by Executive Order, mandated the establishment of the National Center for Bioethics in Research and Heath Care at Tuskegee University. After two years, in 1999, the Bioethics Center opened.

CONTENT

One of the options for the essayists contributing to this book was to critically review the seven articles published by Katz et al.[12] Ideally, the goal of this book and other salient writings related to health equity is to improve the health of underserved populations by better understanding the conditions and circumstance that create ill health. Katz's series of publications targeted two fundamental questions relevant to that goal: Are black people more reluctant than Hispanics or non-Hispanic whites to participate as research subjects in biomedical studies, and does awareness of the "Tuskegee Syphilis Study" lead to reluctance by either of the above listed groups to participate in biomedical studies? Their major findings were that black people are not more reluctant to participate in biomedical research than are Hispanics or non-Hispanic whites. Also, the Tuskegee Syphilis Study was not associated with willingness to participate in biomedical studies either for black people or for non-Hispanic whites. However, they also found that black people and Hispanics had a higher "wariness" about participating than did non-Hispanic whites. They concluded that researchers can successfully comply with the 1994 NIH Guidelines for the Inclusion of Women and Minorities in Biomedical Studies despite the research "abuse horrors, the long-rumored 'legacy' of the Tuskegee Syphilis Study, per se, is not an 'insurmountable issue to overcome; and that despite lower trust levels and historically lower rates of participation, if 'active plans are put into action' diversity in study populations will be achieved." (see the appendix for a list of the seven TLP studies by Katz et al.).[12]

Further, conclusions drawn from the work of Katz et al., conducted some 30 years after the ending of that original study, also provide ample evidence that African Americans' awareness of the so-called Tuskegee Syphilis Study, which was significantly higher than in whites or Hispanics, did not appear to affect blacks' willingness to participate in biomedical studies today, some three decades after "the event." However, if the USPHS Syphilis Study at Tuskegee, in particular, is symbolically and metaphorically used as an example of historical and current injustices in health care, undergirded by human subject research, a broader insight may be revealed. The many instances of injustice and unethical behavior in the health care system are well documented throughout annuals of health and health care in the U.S.[1,13–20] Acknowledging the interconnection between the metaphor of the USPHS Syphilis Study at Tuskegee and the litany of health and health care abuses experienced by black people provide a more in-depth understanding of the "perhaps now invisible" long-term impact of that infamous study. African Americans continue to experience persistent morbidity and mortality, excess deaths, worsening health disparities, continuing environmental injustices, limited geographical and financial access to health care and high health illiteracy rates. Examples include, but are not limited, to the following:

- For the first time, the U.S. federal government documented that morbidity and mortality could be chronicled by race and ethnicity in the 1985 Report of the Secretary's Task Force on Black and Minority Health. Then-Secretary of the Department of Health and Human Services Margret Heckler wrote that "[health] disparity has existed ever since Federal record keeping began more than a generation ago and although our health charts do itemize steady gains in health of minority Americans, the stubborn disparity remains . . . an affront to both our ideas and to the ongoing genius of American medicine." The term excess deaths was used for the first time in the Task Force Report to document the difference between the number of deaths expected if the minority population had the same age and sex-specific death rates as their non-Hispanic white counterparts and reported 60,000 excess deaths among black people in 1985.[14] In 1994, Osler indicated that health disparities were worsening.[21] In 2005, Satcher et al. reported excess deaths among the black population had risen to 83,000.[22] *Black health disparities are worsening!*

- The U.S. Environment Protection Agency has ample evidence on the adverse affects of toxic and hazardous waste on human health.[23] A 1987 report, updated in 1994, published by the Commission for Racial Justice of the United Church of Christ found that communities where racial minority populations lived had significantly more commercial hazardous-waste facilities than communities consisting of non-Hispanic whites regardless of income status.[23] *Environmental injustices continue!*

- Geographic and finical access to health care remains a barrier for many people in the U.S., particularly in urban and rural communities. These communities are disproportionately minority and low income. Many of the 43,000,000 people in the U.S. who are uninsured or underinsured live in these areas.[15] *Unequal treatment in health care delivery remains!*

- The American Medical Association reported that poor health literacy is a "stronger predictor of a person's health than age, income, employment status, education level and race."[24] Ninety million people in the United States alone have difficulty understanding and using health information.[25] *Health equity depends on an array of rights beyond health!*

These problems symbolically all represent a "Tuskegee Syphilis Study episode" because at they are all bioethics and public health ethics violations. Based on the current state of scientific knowledge, these problems are all potentially preventable and their adverse impact can be reduced, if not eliminated.[22] At the core, they are all profoundly wrong.

REFLECTIONS

The metaphoric phrase "sin-sick soul" in this essay's title emphasizes the healing process necessary to reframe the tragedy of the USPHS Syphilis Study at Tuskegee into an opportunity for social justice. Metaphysically, sin is simply a mistake that results in consequence, not punishment. Soul is the subjective side of life that takes the thought of the conscious mind and acts upon it.[26] In *Care of the Soul*, Moore writes, "Soul is not a thing but a quality of experiencing life and ourselves."[27] The USPHS Syphilis Study at Tuskegee will remain an adverse lived experience in the souls of black people until social justice related to health, human subject research, and health care health are realized. Health, in this instance, is not a destination, but a journey to reach one's greatest state of aliveness.[28]

The Context and Content sections of this essay are summarized under two spheres of ethics; bioethics and public health ethics.[29] Symbolically, both sections are segments of the "Tuskegee Syphilis Study" episode that have bioethics and public health ethics violations. At the core there were, "wrongdoings" on the part of the federal government and others that occurred and continue to occur.[5] The bioethical violations were that the men were objects of a morally and scientifically flawed research project, and they were denied health care. The public health ethics violations were that the men were singled out because they were members of a vulnerable demographic group as they were black men of lower socioeconomic status, lesser educated than the general population and living in a small, southern rural community with limited access to health care. In 2010, these same demographics characterize the population that experiences the highest morbidity and mortality rates in the country. Unfortunately, these ethical violations in health and health care are embedded in the cultural experience of black people.[30] The research approach and findings of Katz et al. provide an important step in the healing process as we search for the true "legacy" of this tragic study as conducted by the U.S. government. The next step is to further explore the issue through focus group sessions with a cross section of African Americans. These sessions must start with the surviving family members of the men involved in the USPHS Syphilis Study at Tuskegee, using the "story telling" methodology described by Wimberly's Soul Stories, a model focusing on story linking, which is a process of African Americans connecting components of everyday life stories with the Christian faith story found in biblical Scripture and with African American exemplars, past and present.[31] The Pew Forum has documented that African Americans are the most religious group in the U.S.[32] Culture and religion, particularly among African Americans, are interwoven and interdependent and cannot be separated.[30]

Thus, to respond to the USPHS Syphilis Study at Tuskegee in the cultural context of the African American population, religious experiences of African Americans must also be considered. Wimberly writes that storytelling "reveal[s] the roots of . . . [black] history, aspect[s] of their own experience [as] they live in the present and their hopes for the future.[31] (p. 4). Surely, within its cultural context and content, the legacy of the USPHS Syphilis Study at Tuskegee is in the root of the history—present and future—of African Americans and all people of goodwill. If appropriately addressed the souls of black folks can be cared for, nurtured and healed.[33] Until then, the soul of America will not be at peace.

Rueben C. Warren, DDS, MPH, DrPH, MDiv, is professor and director of the Tuskegee National Center for Bioethics. Adjunct appointments: professor of public health, medicine and ethics, Interdenominational Theological Center; clinical professor, Department of Community Health/Preventive Medicine, Morehouse School of Medicine; professor, Department of Behavioral Sciences and Health Education, Emory's Rollins School of Public Health; and professor, Schools of Dentistry and Graduate Studies, Meharry Medical College. Dr. Warren was associate director for Minority Health, Centers for Disease Control and Prevention. He directed Infrastructure Development, National Center on Minority Health and Health Disparities, NIH. Formerly, he was dean of the Meharry Medical College School of Dentistry.

NOTES

1. Campbell, A. (1995). *Health As Liberation: Medicine, Theology, and the Quest for Justice* Cleveland: The Pilgrim Press.

2. Centers for Disease Control and Prevention.

3. Vonderlehr, R. A., Bundesen, H., Moore, J., Nelson, N. A., Pelouze, P. S., Snow, W. F., Usilton, L. J., et al. (1936). Recommendations for A Venereal Disease Control Program. *Journal of the American Medical Association, 106*(2), 115–118. doi: 10.1001/jama.1936.02770020002049.

4. Reverby, S. (2009). *Examining Tuskegee: The Infamous Syphilis Study and Its Legacy.* Chapel Hill: The University of North Carolina Press.

5. The White House Office of the Press Secretary. (1997). Remarks by the President in apology for study done in Tuskegee. Retrieved December 31st, 2010, from http://clinton4.nara.gov/textonly/New/Remarks/Fri/19970516-898.html.

6. Warren, R., & Tarver, W. L. (2010). A foundation for public health ethics at Tuskegee University in the 21st century. *J Health Care Poor Underserved, 21*(3 Suppl), 46–56. doi: S1548686910300064 (p. ii).

7. Office of Management and Budget (Producer). (1977 November 18th, 2010). Revisions to the Standards for the Classification of Federal Data on Race and Ethnicity *Race Data.* Retrieved from http://www.census.gov/population/www/socdemo/race/Ombdir15.html.

8. Gamble, V. (2010). University Professor of Medical Humanities and Professor of History.

9. Associate Director for Minority Health Office of the Director. (1995). Associate Director for Minority Health Office of the Director Annual Program Briefing Atlanta U.S. Department of Health and Human Services.

10. Jones, J. (1993). *Bad Blood: The Tuskegee Syphilis Experiment (New and Expanded Edition).* New York: The Free Press.

11. See the introduction of this book.

12. Katz, R. V., Kegeles, S. S., Green, B. L., Kressin, N. R., James, S. A., and Claudio, C. (2003). The Tuskegee Legacy Project: history, preliminary scientific findings and unanticipated societal benefits, *Dent Clin of North America* 47(1):1–19.

13. De La Cancela, V., Lau Chin, J., and Jenkins, Y. (1998). *Community Health Psychology* New York Routledge.

14. Department of Health and Human Services. (1985). Black and Minority Health. Report of the Secretary's Task Force. Volume 1: Executive Summary (Vol. 1, pp. 1–244). Washington, D.C.

15. Department of Health and Human Services. (2009). Health, United States, 2009 with Special Feature on Medical Technology Hyattsville National Center for Health Statistics.

16. Institute of Medicine. (2003). Assessing Potential Sources of Racial and Ethnic Disparities in Care: Patient-and System-Level Factors.

17. Walker, B., Mays, V. M., and Warren, R. (2004). The changing landscape for the elimination of racial/ethnic health status disparities. *J Health Care Poor Underserved, 15*(4), 506–521. doi: S1548686904405063 (p. ii).

18. Warren, R. (1992). Health Education and Black Health Status In R. Braithwaite & S. Taylor (Eds.), *Health Issues in the Black Community.* San Francisco: Jossey-Bass.

19. Warren, R. (2001). Enhancing oral and systemic health. *Compend Contin Educ Dent, 22*(3, Spec. No.), 4–11.

20. Washington, H. (2006). *Medical Apartheid: The Dark History of Medical Experimentation on Black Americans from Colonial Times to the Present* New York Doubleday.

21. Osler, W. (1994). Preface. In L. I. Livingston (Ed.), *Handbook of Black American Health: The mosaic of conditions, issues, policies and prospects* Westport: Greenwood Press.

22. Satcher, D., Fryer, G. E., Jr., McCann, J., Troutman, A., Woolf, S. H., & Rust, G. (2005). What if we were equal? A comparison of the black-white mortality gap in 1960 and 2000. *Health Aff (Millwood), 24*(2), 459–464. doi: 24/2/459 (p. ii).

23. Institute of Medicine. (1999). *Toward Environmental Justice: Research, Education, and Health Policy Needs* Washington, D.C.: National Academy Press.

24. American Medical Association. (1999). Health Literacy: Report of the Council on Scientific Affairs. *JAMA, 281*(6), 552–557.

25. Needed Research. In B. Smedley, A. Stith & A. Nelson (Eds.), *Unequal Treatment: Confronting Racial and Ethnic Disparities in Healthcare* (pp. 143–144). Washington, DC: National Academy of Sciences.

26. Holmes, E. (2007). *The Science of Mind* Radford Wilder Publications, LLC.

27. Moore, T. (1992). *Care of the Soul: A Guide for Cultivating Depth and Sacredness in Everyday Life.* New York: HarperPerennial.

28. Chissell, J. T. (1993). *Pyramids of power! An ancient African centered approach to optimal health.* Baltimore: Positive Perceptions Publications.

29. Bayer, R., Gostin, L., and B., J. (2007). *Public Health Ethic: Theory, Policy, and Practice.* New York: Oxford University Press.

30. King, L. (2002). Development of Authenticity in Public Health. In J. C. Chunn (Ed.), *The Health Behavioral Change Imperative: Theory, Eduction, and Practice in Diverse Populations.* New York: Kluwer Academic/Plenum Publishers.

31. Wimberly, A. (2005). *Soul Stories: An African American Christian Education.* Nashville: Abingdon Press.

32. The Pew Forum on Religion and Public Life. (2009). A Religious Portrait of African-Americans, retrieved November 12th 2010, from http://pewforum.org /A-Religious-Portrait-of-African-Americans.aspx.

33. Du Bois, W. E. B. (1903). *The Souls of Black Folk: Essays and Sketches.* Cambridge, MA: John Wilson and Son.

Appendix

The Seven Key Articles from the Tuskegee Legacy Project, as Read by All Essayists

Are minorities more reluctant to participate in biomedical research than whites?

Katz, R. V., Kegeles, S. S., Kressin, N. R., Green, B. L., Wang, M. Q., James S. A., Russell, S. L., and Claudio, C. The Tuskegee Legacy Project: Willingness of Minorities to Participate in Biomedical Research. *J Health Care for the Poor and Underserved* 2006, 17:698–715.

Katz, R. V., Green, B. L., Kressin, N. R., Claudio, C., Wang, M. Q., and Russell, S.L. Willingness of Minorities to Participate in Biomedical Studies: confirmatory findings from a follow-up study using the Tuskegee Legacy Project Questionnaire. *J National Medical Association.* 2007, 99(9): 1050–62.

Does either general awareness or detailed knowledge about the USPHS Syphilis Study at Tuskegee affect willingness to participate in biomedical research?

Katz, R. V., Green, B. L., Kressin, N. R., Kegeles, S. S., Wang, M. Q., James, S. A., Russell, S. L., Claudio, C., and McCallum, J. The Legacy of the Tuskegee Syphilis Study: Its Impact on Willingness to Participate in Biomedical Research Studies. *J Health Care for the Poor and Underserved* 2008, 19:1169–1181.

Katz, R. V., Green, B. L., PhD, Kressin, N. R., James, S. A., Claudio, C., Wang, M. Q., and Russell, S. L. Exploring the "Legacy" of the Tuskegee Syphilis Study: A follow-up study from the Tuskegee Legacy Project. *J National Medical Association.* Feb. 2009: 101(2):179–183.

Does awareness of the Presidential Apology for the USPHS Syphilis Study at Tuskegee influence minority participation in biomedical research?

Katz, R. V., Kegeles, S. S., Kressin, N. R., James, S. A., Green, B. L., Wang, M. Q., Russell, S. L., and Claudio, C. Awareness of the USPHS Syphilis Study at Tuskegee and the U.S. Presidential Apology and Their Influence on Minority Participation in Biomedical Research. *American J Public Health.* 2008, 98:1137–1147.

Is there a difference between minorities and whites in their ability to accurately identify the Tuskegee Syphilis Study?

Katz, R. V., Jean-Charles, G., Green, B. L., Kressin, N. R., Claudio, C., Wang, M. Q., Russell, S. L., and Outlaw, J. Identifying the Tuskegee Syphilis Study: implications of results from recall and recognition questions. *BMC Public Health* 2009, 9:468.

Do minorities, as compared to whites, believe they are "more likely to be taken advantage of" when they participate in biomedical studies or in cancer screenings?

Katz, R. V., Wang, M. Q., Green, B. L., Kressin, N. R., Claudio, C., Russell, S. L., and Sommervil, C. Participation in Biomedical Research Studies and Cancer Screenings: Perceptions of Risks to Minorities Compared with Whites. *Cancer Control* 2008, 15(4) 344–351.

Index

About the Editors and Contributors

Harold L. Aubrey, MS, MURP, EdD (Partner, Sable Investments, LLC), is an applied statistician. In the last 20 years, he has served as a consultant, co-author, or author of over 150 research, evaluation, and planning reports. His primary specialty is the application of advanced statistical methods in the design of experimental and nonexperimental research in education, public health, social sciences, and behavioral sciences. While serving as a higher education administrator (chair, director, assistant dean, dean, assistant vice president, and acting provost) and professor, he has been a chair or committee member of 21 doctoral dissertations.

Ronald L. Braithwaite, PhD, is an educational psychologist and professor in the Departments of Community Health and Preventative Medicine and Psychiatry at Morehouse School of Medicine. He has held faculty appointments at Virginia Commonwealth University, Hampton University, Howard University, Rollins School of Public Health of Emory University, and the School of Public Health at the University of Cape Town, South Africa. His research involves HIV intervention studies with juveniles and adults in correctional systems, social determinants of health, health disparities, and community capacity building. His research spans the globe to Africa, where he has conducted HIV-prevention projects.

Virginia Brennan, PhD, MA, has been the editor of the *Journal of Health Care for the Poor and Underserved* since 2001. She is a member of the faculty of Meharry Medical College. She is the editor of and a contributor to the book *Natural Disasters and Public Health: Hurricanes Katrina, Rita, and Wilma* (Johns Hopkins University Press, 2009) and of another book (on free clinics) scheduled for publication in Winter 2011/2012. She was previously a faculty member in linguistics and psychology at Swarthmore College and Vanderbilt University.

Giselle Corbie-Smith, MD, MSc (professor, Departments of Social Medicine and Medicine, UNC–Chapel Hill), is a clinician researcher who directs the Program on Health Disparities at the Sheps Center and the Community Engagement Core of the NC Translational and Clinical Sciences Institute. She is nationally recognized for her scholarly work on practical and ethical issues of involving communities of color in research and has served on numerous local, regional and national committees.

Mario De La Rosa, PhD, is a professor at the Robert Stemple College of Public Health and Social Work, Florida International University (FIU). He received his doctorate from Ohio State University and has published more than 80 scholarly publications on Latino substance abuse and HIV and other underserved populations. His career is highlighted by his effort to bring about a reduction in health disparities in our nation by working together with other researchers across the country. Dr. De La Rosa has also received funding from NIH on numerous occasions and served on numerous national scientific review panels and advisory councils.

Riggins R. Earl Jr., BA, MDiv, PhD (professor of ethics and theology, Interdenominational Theological Center Atlanta), is an ethicist who has focused his research, writing, and teaching on the ethical life of blacks in America. Earl seeks to show how the experiences of racism, classicism and genderism, as expressed through slavery and segregation, framed the context for blacks' ethical responses; his book on this theme is *Dark Symbols, Obscure Signs: God, Self, and Community in the Slave Mind.* Having published an article on the ethics of the Tuskegee Syphilis Study, he is now writing a book on that topic.

M. Joycelyn Elders, MD, MS (professor emeritus of pediatrics and public health at UAMS), was the 15th US Surgeon General, serving under President Bill Clinton. She also has been the director of the Arkansas Department of Health, president of ASTHO, member of the IRB at UAMS for seven years, and served on multiple NIH and FDA Advisory Committees. She is currently a member of multiple medical organizations and presently serves as co-chair of the Trojan Sexual Health Advisory Committee. She is a pediatric endocrinologist and was a researcher primarily in the areas of growth and development and public health, with extensive publications.

James P. Griffin Jr., PhD (research associate professor in the Department of Community Health and Preventive Medicine at Morehouse School of Medicine), is trained in community and organizational psychology. Much of his work has been in collaboration with community-based organizations including violence-, substance abuse–, HIV-, and hepatitis-prevention initiatives. He also has experience providing programs for inmates returning to the community. His NIH-funded substance abuse and violence prevention program was career- and resiliency-based and involved African American males. He is the founder and convener of the Metropolitan Atlanta Violence Prevention Partnership (MAVPP) and recipient of multiple community service awards.

Malika Roman Isler, PhD, MPH (research assistant professor of social medicine, UNC Chapel Hill School of Medicine), is a social scientist who has focused on socio-cultural constructions of health and models of community partnership in research. As the assistant director of the NC Translational and Clinical Sciences Institute Community Engagement Core, she facilitates community-based research infrastructures and capacity building to support community-academic partnerships in translational research. Her primary research focuses on community engagement in HIV prevention, HIV technology trials, population-based genomics initiatives, and access to HIV clinical trials.

James H. Jones, PhD (alumni distinguished professor, emeritus, University of Arkansas), is an American social and intellectual historian who specializes in the history of science and medicine. In addition to *Bad Blood: The Tuskegee Syphilis Experiment*, he is the author of *Alfred C. Kinsey, A Public/ Private Life*. His essays and book reviews have appeared in *The New Yorker*, the *New York Times*, the *Washington Post*, and the *Los Angeles Times*. He lives in Washington, D.C.

Ralph V. Katz, DMD, MPH, PhD (professor and chair, Department of Epidemiology & Health Promotion, NYU College of Dentistry), is an epidemiologist who has focused on oral diseases and health disparities and has led the Tuskegee Legacy Project research study team since 1997. He served as the director of two NIH-funded oral health research centers focused on health disparities and minority health between 1992 and 2009. Having served on the National Legacy Committee which initiated the formal request for a Presidential Apology, he was an invitee to the White House by President Clinton for the May 1997 Presidential Apology for the Tuskegee Syphilis Study.

R. L'Heureux Lewis, PhD (assistant professor, Department of Sociology and Black Studies Program, the City College of New York–CUNY), is a sociologist who focuses on issues of race and ethnicity. His work concentrates on African American education, health, and gender relations. His major line of research explores how inequality is structured and how policy responses can reduce these inequalities. He is the author of the forthcoming book *Inequality in the Promised Land: New Dilemmas in Race, Education and Opportunity*. He was selected as a Ford Foundation Diversity Fellow and an American Sociological Association Mental Health Minority Fellow.

Vickie M. Mays, *Ph.D., MSPH* (Professor of Psychology and Health Services, UCLA), is a clinical psychologist trained in health services and epidemiology who has published papers on research ethics in racial/ethnic minority populations. Funded by a NIH T32, she created a course on research ethics in behavioral and biomedical research in racial/ethnic minorities. Her interests in research ethics include HIV/AIDS, ethics of research methodologies, data policies, and data analytic strategies in working with African Americans and small-sample populations such as American Indians. She is the director of the Center on Health Policy and Minority Health Disparities.

Mary E. Northridge, PhD, MPH, is editor-in-chief of the *American Journal of Public Health* and was professor of Clinical Sociomedical Sciences (in dental medicine) at the Columbia University Mailman School of Public Health at the time of this research and writing, where she still holds a part-time appointment. She is currently in the Department of Epidemiology and Health Promotion at the NYU College of Dentistry. Professor Northridge has enduring interests in social and environmental determinants of health, including oral health, and an emerging focus in the utility of systems science to integrate and sustain holistic health and health care for older adults.

Adebowale A. Odulana, MD, MPH (NRSA Primary Care Research Fellow at the Sheps Center for Health Services Research at UNC–Chapel Hill), is trained in internal medicine and pediatrics, with research interests in health disparities and pediatric obesity. He is currently working on research projects aimed at reducing minority health disparities through church-based participatory research and projects evaluating medical decision aids in relation to African American men.

Vivian W. Pinn, MD, is director of the Office of Research on Women's Health of the National Institutes of Health. Prior to NIH, she was professor and chair of pathology at Howard University College of Medicine after faculty appointments at Tufts and Harvard medical schools. As past-president of the National Medical Association and in her role at the NIH, she has long been active in efforts to address health disparities and encourage the participation of minorities and women in research. She was invited to the White House for President Clinton's May 1997 Presidential Apology for the Tuskegee Syphilis Study.

Susan M. Reverby, PhD (McLean Professor in the History of Ideas and professor of women's and gender studies, Wellesley College) is a historian of American women, nursing, race, and health care. Her books include her edited *Tuskegee's Truths: Rethinking the Tuskegee Syphilis Study* (2000) and her prize-winning *Examining Tuskegee: The Infamous Syphilis Study and its Legacy* (2009). She was a member of the Legacy Committee that organized for a federal apology for the study. Her most recent article on the PHS's inoculation STD studies in Guatemala led to worldwide media attention and another apology from the White House.

David Satcher, MD, PhD, and director of The Satcher Health Leadership Institute established in 2006 at the Morehouse School of Medicine in Atlanta, Georgia, was sworn in as the 16th surgeon general of the United States in 1998. His tenure of public service includes serving as director of the Centers for Disease Control and Prevention (CDC). He was the first person to have served as Director of the CDC and then surgeon general of the United States. Dr. Satcher has also held top leadership positions at the Charles R. Drew University for Medicine and Science and the Meharry Medical College.

Rueben C. Warren, DDS, MPH, DrPH, MDiv, is professor and director of the Tuskegee National Center for Bioethics. Adjunct appointments: professor of public health, medicine, and ethics, Interdenominational Theological Center; clinical professor, Department of Community Health/Preventive Medicine, Morehouse School of Medicine; professor, Department of Behavioral Sciences and Health Education, Emory's Rollins School of Public Health; and professor, Schools of Dentistry and Graduate Studies, Meharry Medical College. Dr. Warren was associate director for Minority Health, Centers for Disease Control and Prevention. He directed Infrastructure Development, National Center on Minority Health and Health Disparities, NIH. Formerly he was dean of the Meharry Medical College School of Dentistry.

Luther S. Williams, PhD (distinguished professor of biology, dean of graduate studies and research, and provost and vice president for academic affairs, Tuskegee University), is a molecular biologist whose basic research has focused on the control of gene expression for the majority of his 41-year career. More recently his work has addressed underrepresentation of minorities in science and engineering and he presently directs a NIH-funded bioethics infrastructure initiative focused on bioethics training. He has served as a member of the National Center (Institute) for Minority Health Disparities Advisory Council and currently serves as a member of the NIH Director's Council.

Monique M. Williams, MD, MSCI (assistant professor of medicine and psychiatry, Division of Geriatrics and Nutritional Science, Washington University School of Medicine), serves as the director of the African American Outreach Satellite, Knight Alzheimer's Disease Research Center, and Community Outreach and Recruitment Core of the NIH-funded Bioethics Infrastructure Initiative. Her principal research foci are Alzheimer's disease in African Americans and minority participation in clinical trials.

CPSIA information can be obtained at www.ICGtesting.com
Printed in the USA

269520BV00004B/7/P